Praise for
Fostering a Research-Intensive Organization

"This book is a wealth of insights into how to create and sustain a culture of inquiry within healthcare organizations, where evidence-based decisions are fundamental to safe and effective healthcare. Great examples are offered in every chapter on how to engage clinical care nurses in research and its applications. Find out from this book how your organization can create a culture that values and acts upon research evidence."

—Linda H. Aiken, PhD, RN, FAAN, FRCN
Professor and Director, Center for Health Outcomes and Policy Research
University of Pennsylvania School of Nursing

"This extraordinary resource chronicles the Massachusetts General Hospital interdisciplinary journey to scientific inquiry and discovery leading to evidence-based practice changes that improve patient outcomes. This book will serve as a guide for nursing organizations, scientists, and nurse mentors in developing their own programs of research. A timely resource for now and the new healthcare age of rapid transformation."

—Mary Gullatte, PhD, RN, ANP-BC, AOCN, FAAN
Corporate Director of Nursing Innovation and Research, EMORY Healthcare

"On any day at Massachusetts General Hospital, the breadth of nursing research is evident in the breadth of research presentations and bedside quality innovations. Ives Erickson, Jones, Ditomassi, and colleagues have created a culture that encourages inquiry, requires evidence, and measures outcomes. In their new book, *Fostering a Research-Intensive Organization: An Interdisciplinary Approach for Nurses From Massachusetts General Hospital*, we see the underpinnings of a local strategy that has become a national model."

—Karen Donelan, ScD, EdM
Senior Scientist in Health Policy, Mongan Institute for Health Policy,
Massachusetts General Hospital
Adjunct Faculty, Center for Interdisciplinary Health Workforce Studies,
Vanderbilt University School of Medicine

"This is a one-of-a-kind presentation of the origins and operations of a carefully developed set of initiatives to advance nursing scholarship and scholarly nursing practice in one of the world's premier academic health sciences centers. It will surely provide much inspiration for nurse leaders and researchers on the lookout for new ways to leverage the unique opportunities to bring together people, ideas, and resources in practice settings to develop and translate nursing knowledge."

–*Sean Clarke, PhD, RN, FAAN*
Professor and Associate Dean
Connell School of Nursing, Boston College

"This book provides an excellent blueprint for those who want to take nursing practice to the next level. The creation of a culture of inquiry that is synchronized with a nursing research agenda is one illustration of how this book provides a detailed path for restructuring that can improve and enhance the nursing experience and, most importantly, patient care delivery."

–*Bonnie B. Blanchfield, ScD, CPA*
Senior Scientist in Health Policy, Mongan Institute for Health Policy,
Massachusetts General Hospital

Fostering a Research-Intensive Organization

An Interdisciplinary Approach for Nurses From Massachusetts General Hospital

Jeanette Ives Erickson, DNP, RN, NEA-BC, FAAN
Marianne Ditomassi, DNP, MBA, RN
Dorothy A. Jones, EdD, RN, FAAN, FNI

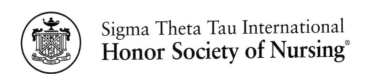

Sigma Theta Tau International
Honor Society of Nursing®

The Honor Society of Nursing, Sigma Theta Tau International (STTI) is a nonprofit organization founded in 1922 whose mission is advancing world health and celebrating nursing excellence in scholarship, leadership, and service. Members include practicing nurses, instructors, researchers, policymakers, entrepreneurs, and others. STTI's 499 chapters are located at more than 695 institutions of higher education throughout Australia, Botswana, Brazil, Canada, Colombia, Ghana, Hong Kong, Japan, Kenya, Malawi, Mexico, the Netherlands, Pakistan, Portugal, Singapore, South Africa, South Korea, Swaziland, Sweden, Taiwan, Tanzania, United Kingdom, United States, and Wales. More information about STTI can be found online at www.nursingsociety.org.

Sigma Theta Tau International
550 West North Street
Indianapolis, IN, USA 46202

To order additional books, buy in bulk, or order for corporate use, contact Nursing Knowledge International at 888.NKI.4YOU (888.654.4968/US and Canada) or +1.317.634.8171 (outside US and Canada).

To request a review copy for course adoption, email solutions@nursingknowledge.org or call 888.NKI.4YOU (888.654.4968/US and Canada) or +1.317.634.8171 (outside US and Canada).

To request author information, or for speaker or other media requests, contact Marketing, Honor Society of Nursing, Sigma Theta Tau International at 888.634.7575 (US and Canada) or +1.317.634.8171 (outside US and Canada).

ISBN: 9781940446004
EPUB ISBN: 9781940446011
PDF ISBN: 9781940446028
MOBI ISBN: 9781940446035

Library of Congress Cataloging-in-Publication Data

Ives Erickson, Jeanette, author.
  Fostering a research-intensive organization : an interdisciplinary approach for nurses from Massachusetts General Hospital / Jeanette Ives Erickson, Marianne Ditomassi, Dorothy Jones.
      p. ; cm.
  Includes bibliographical references.
  ISBN 978-1-940446-00-4 (print : alk. paper) -- ISBN 978-1-940446-01-1 (epub) -- ISBN 978-1-940446-02-8 (pdf) -- ISBN 978-1-940446-03-5 (mobi)
  I. Ditomassi, Marianne, author. II. Jones, Dorothy A., author. III. Sigma Theta Tau International, issuing body. IV. Title.
  [DNLM: 1. Massachusetts General Hospital. 2. Nursing Research--methods--Massachusetts. 3. Evidence-Based Nursing--methods--Massachusetts. 4. Hospitals, General--Massachusetts. 5. Models, Nursing--Massachusetts. 6. Program Development--methods--Massachusetts. WY 20.5]
  RT81.5
  610.73072--dc23
                          2015014962

First Printing, 2015

Publisher: Dustin Sullivan
Acquisitions Editor: Emily Hatch
Editorial Coordinator: Paula Jeffers
Cover Designer: Michael Tanamachi
Interior Design/Page Layout: Kim Scott

Principal Book Editor: Carla Hall
Development and Project Editor: Rebecca Senninger
Copy Editor: Keith Cline
Proofreader: Kevin Kent
Indexer: Larry Sweazy

Dedication

This book is dedicated to our parents and the nurses who have shaped us in our careers. They provided us with the values that guided us to the profession of nursing and allowed us the precious opportunity to advance an environment that is built upon a spirit of inquiry. These values and this passion for nursing have led to our shared commitment. We are grateful to all who believe in the profession of nursing.

Acknowledgments

"I think one's feelings waste themselves in words; they ought all to be distilled into actions, and into actions which bring results."

–Florence Nightingale

Preparing this book has been a labor of love allowing the editors to reflect on the importance of nursing research and the importance of application of evidence-based practice especially within the practice environment. The editors are extremely grateful to nurses from around the world, especially those at the Massachusetts General Hospital who deliver high-quality care in the many settings where nursing care is delivered. Thank you for your spirit of inquiry, for your thoughtful innovation, and for caring.

To the many leaders and nurse researchers who have inspired each of us to do our best: Your generosity of spirit, knowledge, and time guides us to continuously advance our practice and our careers, dedicating ourselves to the growth of the discipline and the ultimate good of patient care.

Jeanette Ives Erickson is especially thankful to her family, who has always guided and supported her. To Muriel Poulin, Yvonne Munn, Dorothy A. Jones, and Edward Coakley, faculty who support the MGH and MGH clinicians, who advance the art and science of nursing, I will be forever in your debt, as you shared your love of nursing and were always helping me to be a better nurse and leader. The influence of the incredible nurses, health professionals, support staff, and physicians that I have had the pleasure of working with throughout my career will always be a special part of who I am. You have always challenged me, given me great joy, and made me proud to work side by side with you. Massachusetts General Hospital has provided me a strong foundation for future innovations that I hope will benefit those we serve.

Marianne Ditomassi is appreciative for the support and mentorship she has received from her family, from teachers, and from colleagues throughout her career, including Jeanette Ives Erickson, Dorothy A. Jones, Ann Minnick, and

Marilyn Neuman. Your belief and trust in me have enabled me to have a career and life full of creativity, influence, and learning.

Dorothy A. Jones is forever grateful for her family, who gives her the freedom "to be and become." In addition, she is also thankful for the presence of nurse leaders such as Dorothy DeMaio, Mary Duffy, Marjory Gordon, Trish Gibbons, Catherine Murphy, and Margaret Newman in her life. These inspirational nurses have led the development of nursing knowledge and have guided Dorothy in her pursuit of nursing knowledge, the delivery of quality patient care, and the search for truth through inquiry. To colleagues I have worked with and students I have taught past and present at Boston University and Boston College, William F. Connell School of Nursing. Thank you. You have transformed my life.

We also acknowledge Massachusetts General Hospital and its leadership and researchers who have led the academic mission locally, nationally, and internationally.

About the Authors

Jeanette Ives Erickson, DNP, RN, NEA-BC, FAAN

Jeanette Ives Erickson is Chief Nurse and Senior Vice President for Patient Care Services at Massachusetts General Hospital (MGH); Instructor at Harvard Medical School; Assistant Professor at the Massachusetts General Hospital Institute of Health Professions; Chairperson of the Board of the Lunder-Dineen Health Education Alliance of Maine; and Westbrook College Alumni Trustee on the University of New England Board of Trustees. As chief nurse and senior vice president, she is responsible for clinical practice, research, education, and community service, serving 5,300 nurses, health professionals, and support staff.

While fostering nursing research within an interdisciplinary, professional practice model, Ives Erickson has built upon the vision of her predecessor, Yvonne L. Munn, RN, MS (1984–1993), who valued nursing research and hoped to infuse it into the fabric of patient care at the MGH. Over the years, Ives Erickson has worked to advance a research agenda, which has become an integral component of nursing and collaborative practice. The development of the Yvonne L. Munn Center, within the Institute for Patient Care, has become an important vehicle to generate, translate, and utilize nursing knowledge to enhance patient care and professional development.

Ives Erickson has been a participant in the development of measures to evaluate professional practice, has participated in multiple presentations, and has been the lead author on publications that facilitate the dissemination of multiple research initiatives at the MGH. She has presented globally and consults on multiple issues affecting nurse autonomy, leadership development, collaborative decision-making, and Magnet® hospital recognition.

Marianne Ditomassi, DNP, MBA, RN

Marianne Ditomassi is Executive Director of Patient Care Services operations at Massachusetts General Hospital (MGH), which supports the work of the senior vice president for patient care and chief nurse, who oversees the operations of nursing, the therapy departments and social services. Her key areas of accountability include strategic planning, recruitment and retention initiatives, business planning, fundraising, and communications. In addition, she is the Magnet program director for MGH and successfully coordinated MGH's initial Magnet Recognition Program® journey in 2003 and subsequent Magnet® re-designations in 2008 and 2013.

Prior to her current roles, Ditomassi served as founding director of the Center for Clinical and Professional Development at MGH. During her leadership in this position, she launched a department that focused on translating the professional practice model for nursing and other health professions into reality. She is a graduate of Georgetown University and Loyola University in Chicago, Illinois, for her undergraduate and graduate degrees in nursing, respectively, and of University of Illinois for her graduate degree in business. She received her doctorate of nursing practice degree in executive practice from the MGH Institute of health professions.

Dorothy A. Jones EdD, RN, FAAN, FNI

Dorothy A. Jones is the current Director and Senior Nurse Scientist in the Yvonne L. Munn Center for Nursing Research and Professor of Nursing at Boston College William F. Connell School of Nursing. As the first director of the Munn Center, Jones brings to her work a vision of the potential research and inquiry have on expanding nursing's visibility as a significant contributor to patient care through research. Jones is an author of multiple books and over 135 international publications. She is the recipient of many awards and honors and is a funded researcher by external groups including NIH-NINR. Jones has worked closely with Jeanette Ives Erickson and Marianne Ditomassi to develop the infrastructure essential to the advancement of patient care through nursing research.

The Munn Center is one of four centers within the Institute for Patient Care. Since its inception in 2006, it has gained global recognition as a setting that is able to promote a nursing research agenda within the culture of clinical practice. Jones has a history of organizational leadership serving as president of NANDA International and the Eastern Nursing Research Society. She has served in academic leadership roles and holds a visiting professorship at the University of Navarra and the Clinica Universitas in Pamplona, Spain. She actively participates in the conduct of multisite research in areas including workforce evaluation, symptom management, and transition care, theory development and research within Newman's framework of Health as Expanding Consciousness, and has facilitated the development of multiple instruments grounded in qualitative methods. Jones works with many students and staff and nurse scholars on research initiatives and dissertations to advance nursing science and improve patient care.

Contributing Authors

Jeffrey M. Adams, PhD, RN

Jeffrey M. Adams is the Associate Director of the Center for Innovations in Care Delivery, an American Nurses Credentialing Center (ANCC) Scholar, a Connell Research Scholar, and an affiliated faculty of the Mongan Institute for Health Policy at Massachusetts General Hospital (MGH). He is a Visiting Scholar at both the MIT Institute for Soldier Nanotechnologies and Boston College William F. Connell School of Nursing. His interests stem from his experience spanning practice, research, education, policy, and theory emphasizing how nurse leader influence, innovation, and informatics impact professional practice environments and outcomes in healthcare settings across the United States. In 2014, Adams was selected as a Robert Wood Johnson Foundation – Executive Nurse Fellow. He was also recently profiled in the *Journal of Nursing Administration* as the first in a series of emerging administration and policy specialists and in a *Nursing Administration Quarterly* article focused on leadership talent. Adams has developed two published models that guide his work: The Adams Influence Model (AIM) defines the factors, attributes, and process of influence and power; and The Model of the Interrelationship of Leadership, Environments, and Outcomes for Nurse Executives (MILE ONE) synthesizes existing literature to provide structure of emphasis for nursing administration education and care delivery roles. His recently developed instrument measures the Leadership Influence over Professional Practice Environments. One of his current studies using the LIPPES instrument is funded by the ANCC through the American Nurses Foundation and the Connell Family Foundation for use in more than 30 acute care sites throughout the United States. Adams is coordinating efforts at MGH to identify and evaluate innovation in care delivery, and his research in this area suggests mechanisms for accelerating innovation in care delivery. He is on the editorial advisory board of the *Journal of Nursing Administration,* and *The International Journal of Nursing Knowledge and Military Medicine.* Adams writes a recurring column for *JONA* focused on Nurse Leader Influence. He is a Board Member of NANDA-I and an active member of the American Organization of Nurse

Executives, the Organization of Nurse Leaders – Massachusetts/ Rhode Island, and the National Multiple Sclerosis Society. Adams is the author of one book, several book chapters, and multiple peer-reviewed publications and presentations. His educational credentials include a Bachelor of Science in Nursing from the University of Michigan, a Master of Science in Nursing Administration from the University of Pennsylvania, a PhD from Boston College William F. Connell School of Nursing, Postdoctoral Fellowship training at The Massachusetts General Hospital's Yvonne L. Munn Center for Nursing Research, and he has recently completed a Certificate in Applied Biostatistics from Harvard.

Gaurdia Banister, PhD, RN, FAAN

Gaurdia Banister is the executive director of the Institute for Patient Care at Massachusetts General Hospital. The Institute serves as a catalyst for promoting interdisciplinary research, education, and clinical practice development. The ultimate goal of the Institute is to advance the delivery of patient and family centered care by supporting an exemplary practice environment for nurses and members of the health professions. Prior to accepting this position, Banister served as senior vice president for Patient Care Services and Chief Nurse at Providence Hospital, a metropolitan community hospital in Washington, DC, serving the poor and underrepresented populations. Most recently, Banister has academic appointments at the MGH Institute for Health Professions, the William F. Connell School of Nursing at Boston College, and the University of Massachusetts of Boston, College of Nursing and Health Sciences. Banister is a former Johnson and Johnson Wharton Nurse Fellow and an alumna of the Robert Wood Johnson Executive Nurse Fellows Program. Her research interests include innovative models of interprofessional education, transition to practice considerations for culturally diverse nursing students, and the impact of mentoring on career success and progression. She was selected as the Fay W. Whitney School of Nursing distinguished alumna and in 2014 the distinguished alumna for the University of Wyoming, where she received her bachelor's in nursing. She was also chosen as a distinguished alumna at the University of Texas at Austin where she earned both her master's and doctoral degrees. Banister was named as the recipient of the American Nurses Association Mary Eliza Mahoney Award and the Prism Award by the American Organization of the Nurse Executives for her outstanding achievements and leadership in promoting the integration, retention, and advancement of minorities in nursing. Banister is also a Fellow in the American Academy of Nursing.

Howard T. Blanchard, MEd, MS, RN, ACNS-BC, CEN

Howard "Tom" Blanchard is the Clinical Nurse Specialist of the Knight Center for Cardiovascular Therapy at Massachusetts General Hospital's Institute for Heart Vascular and Stroke Care. He serves on hospital-wide interdisciplinary teams, such as the STEMI Quality Committee that brings together nurses, physicians, and administrators from Quality and Safety, the emergency department, and the Catheterization Laboratory to improve the care of patients suffering S-T segment Elevation Myocardial Infarctions. Blanchard works with others to implement programs, such as transitioning from paper-based charting to a hospital system–wide electronic charting. This has involved a number of smaller steps, as well as collaboration among catheterization labs in three hospitals within the system, to refine a charting tool for electronic documentation. Blanchard routinely presents to groups within the hospital, and has spoken to national and international groups on evidence-based practice subjects. Blanchard earned his master's of science in Adult Health Nursing from Boston College, and also earned a master's of education from Boston College. He is a Massachusetts APRN, licensed as a Clinical Nurse Specialist, an Adult Clinical Nurse Specialist - Board Certified, and a Board Certified Emergency Nurse. Blanchard was in the first group to participate in the Clinical Inquiry Institute, a program of Retooling for Evidence-Based Practice (EBP), funded by Health Resources and Services Administration (HRSA) to advance evidence-based practice at MGH. Within this program, he received training in EBP from Marita Titler, PhD, RN, FAAN, and is one of 20 CNS EBP mentors at MGH. Blanchard served on a Massachusetts Department of Public Health stroke report committee for 2 years. He is the immediate past chair of the American Heart Association's Boston Cardiovascular Nursing Education Committee, currently serving as co-chair for planning the 2016 Boston Conference on Cardiovascular Nursing.

Diane L. Carroll, PhD, RN, FAAN

Diane L. Carroll is a Nurse Scientist in the Yvonne L. Munn Center for Nursing Research at Massachusetts General Hospital. Previously, Carroll was the Yvonne L. Munn Nurse Research for 7 years, and a Cardiovascular Clinical Nurse Specialist for 16 years. Carroll was the advisor to the Research and Evidence-Based Practice Committee, a part of the Collaborative Governance at Massachusetts General Hospital. In addition, she chaired a Human Research Committee panel at Partners HealthCare for 10 years. Carroll received her BSN and PhD from Boston College and a master's degree from Salem State University. She is an adjunct Associate Professor at Northeastern University and a Visiting Scholar at Boston College. Carroll maintains programs of research in cardio-vascular nursing and patient safety. She has had regional and national funding for her research. She has over 80 publications in international peer-reviewed journals and has presented her research at a number of national and interna-tional research conferences. In addition to her own program of research, she has mentored 13 staff nurse research studies that were based in clinical practice. Twelve of these studies have been published in peer-reviewed journals. Carroll is currently on the Board of Directors of Eastern Nursing Research Society. She is on the Editorial Board of *Heart & Lung* and *Clinical Pathways in Cardiology*. She is a Nurse Fellow in the European Society of Cardiology, and a Fellow of the American Heart Association and the American Academy of Nursing.

Mary E. Duffy, PhD, RN, FAAN

Mary E. Duffy is currently a Senior Nurse Scientist in the Yvonne L. Munn Center for Nursing Research at Massachusetts General Hospital and Professor Emerita and former Director of the Center for Nursing Research in the William F. Connell School of Nursing at Boston College. She earned her BSN from Villanova University, her MS in Psychiatric Nursing from Rutgers University, and her PhD with a major in nursing from New York University. She is a fel-low in the American Academy of Nursing. In addition to serving as Principal Investigator and Co-Investigator on numerous National Institutes of Health and privately funded projects, Duffy has published extensively throughout her career.

The majority of her publications focus on descriptive and experimental clinical research, instrument development, and psychometric evaluation and on methodological issues in various types of research design. Her current scholarship is focused on advancing nursing knowledge through instrument development and validation research to improve the care of patients and their caregivers.

Jane M. Flanagan, PhD, ANP-BC

Jane M. Flanagan is an Associate Professor and the Program Director of the Adult Gerontology Graduate Program at Boston College William F. Connell School of Nursing. She has appointments as a Nurse Scientist at the Massachusetts General Hospital (MGH), Yvonne L. Munn Center. Flanagan is the Editor for the *International Journal of Nursing Knowledge*. She serves on the Board of Directors in the International Association of Human Caring (IAHC) and as the President for the Society of Rogerian Scholars. Flanagan is a Board Certified Adult Nurse Practitioner who coordinates the Nurses Improving Care for Hospitalized Elders (NICHE) program at MGH. Flanagan earned her BSN from the University of Massachusetts Lowell, her MS from Northeastern University, and her PhD from Boston College. She has authored or co-authored numerous peer-reviewed publications, editorials, and book chapters. She has received external funding from specialty organizations to support her work on patients' response to the illness experience and presented her findings at local, regional, national, and international conferences.

Sara E. Dolan Looby, PhD, ANP-BC, FAAN

Sara E. Dolan Looby is a Nurse Scientist at the Yvonne L. Munn Center for Nursing Research, a Nurse Practitioner in the Program in Nutritional Metabolism within the Neuroendocrine Unit at the Massachusetts General Hospital, and an Assistant Professor of Medicine at Harvard Medical School. At the Munn Center, Looby provides mentorship to staff nurses interested in designing and implementing research projects, abstract development, and dissemination activities including publication. Looby serves on the Partners Institutional Review Board and is co-chair of the Nursing Doctoral Forum, a committee comprising of doctorally prepared nurses at MGH. Additionally, Looby is a reviewer for both nursing and interdisciplinary journals and serves on the Editorial Board of the *Journal of the Association of Nurses in AIDS Care.*

In addition to her activities at the Munn Center, Looby is a member of an established interdisciplinary research team at the MGH Program in Nutritional Metabolism. Looby's program of research includes investigating metabolic complications associated with HIV including osteoporosis, cardiovascular disease, and specifically, co-morbidities and symptoms associated with menopause among women living with HIV. Looby has received independent funding from the NIH, the Harvard Center for AIDS Research, and the Harvard Catalyst. She has numerous publications in a variety of peer-reviewed journals and has presented her research both nationally and internationally. Looby is also a dedicated volunteer health educator at a number of AIDS service organizations throughout Massachusetts and has received many community awards in this regard. Looby obtained her BSN from the University of Vermont, her MSN from the MGH Institute of Health Professions, and her PhD from Boston College. She is a dedicated clinician and researcher who is passionate about improving patient care and quality of life through education and research.

Table of Contents

Foreword

Meaningful Scholarship:
The Hallmark of Clinical Practice

I spent the major portion of my career in academia, largely because that was the arena where I saw the greatest opportunity for innovation and meaningful scholarship when I was starting out as a nurse. Now I'm not so sure that academe is the most dynamic place to be. The emphasis in clinical practice is increasingly on continuous learning, and this stress on developing more nimble healthcare systems has meant that innovation and meaningful scholarship are fast becoming the hallmarks of clinical practice. It is this shift in where the action is that makes this new book on the experience of Massachusetts General Hospital (MGH) so timely, because it recounts how the nurses there moved boldly to enable the real-time generation and application of knowledge for care improvement.

This book is a blueprint of sorts describing how cutting-edge nurses can be in practice settings. There are so many regulatory expectations and trends, from the requirements for qualifying for Magnet® recognition status to the quality improvement push of CMS reimbursement, that require nurses in the practice arena to be on the forefront of translational science. How do we bridge the divide between interventions proven to be efficacious under controlled conditions and apply them in real-life practice so we achieve more effective, higher quality care? And it is a joy to read about what the MGH nurses have successfully accomplished in this direction through their Institute for Patient Care with its four centers aimed at (a) Patient and Family Learning, (b) Nursing Research, (c) Innovations in Care Delivery, and (d) Clinical and Professional Development.

At a time when clinicians must be mindful of best practices and population-based treatment strategies, this book demonstrates how a practice setting can take the lead in developing a culture of inquiry by tackling the issues of the day: for example, the visionary research agenda that a dynamic chief nurse executive can set in motion; the synergistic partnerships that can exist between schools of nursing and nursing services; the role that doctorally prepared nurses can play in significantly improving practice; the changing nature of professional development in academic health centers; and the impact of the electronic health record on nursing research. This book also provides concrete examples of strategies and mechanisms that other practice settings might consider to increase the visibility of nursing research—research awards for staff nurses, pre/post-doctoral support, doctoral forums, workforce evaluation surveys and innovation measures, common patient problems surveys, nursing research grand rounds, multidisciplinary collaborations, international post-doctoral fellows, external nursing faculty scholars and appointments, grant development and mentoring, scholarship and publications, and a dedicated research-focused website.

Twenty-first-century nursing cannot be limited by dated 20th century mindsets, and this volume points the way to new directions where formal evaluation of nursing outcomes is built into the organizational fabric; nurses are sought-after interprofessional team members; proven nursing measures/services are patented and processes licensed; nurses serve as principal investigators for major studies funded by external sources and philanthropic dollars; and the refereed presentations and publications of nurses prove to be the best marketing strategy for recruiting new nurses and convincing patients to choose a particular healthcare system for their needs. Institute of Medicine reports (2003, 2010) have repeatedly called on nurses to exert transformational leadership within healthcare systems, and the MGH nurses are doing just that.

Angela Barron McBride, PhD, RN, FAAN, FNAP
Distinguished Professor-University Dean Emerita,
Indiana University School of Nursing
Board Member, Indiana University Health

References

Institute of Medicine (IOM). (2003). *Keeping patients safe: Transforming the work environment of nurses.* Washington, DC: The National Academies Press.

Institute of Medicine (IOM). (2010). *The future of nursing: Leading change, advancing health.* Washington, DC: The National Academies Press.

Introduction

Implementing a Nursing Research Agenda Within the Clinical Practice Environment

The advancement of nursing research outside of the academic environment continues to grow but its evolution is often challenged by the demands of practice environment. For nurse scientists as well as clinicians, immediate response to patients and their families must take precedence over other professional activities like the pursuit of inquiry. While there is a growing presence of nurse researchers committed to advancing a research agenda within the practice setting, there is often a lack of resources and organizational support to sustain the effort. It is not unusual to have a hospital hire several nurses to lead research initiatives only to find that promoting a culture of inquiry within the practice environment is met with limited resources and time to move work forward.

At the Massachusetts General Hospital, a cohort of more than 50 doctorally prepared nurses as well as staff at the bedside are dedicated to building nursing science and generating and translating evidence to improve practice. The Yvonne L. Munn Center for Nursing Research has helped create an environment dedicated to inquiry for all clinicians and together staff and scholars to actively participate in discovery. These activities have resulted in funding opportunities, new partnerships, enhanced mentoring, and scholarship dedicated to supporting the implementation of a research agenda that addresses the concerns of the discipline. Healthcare reform, changing demographics, and regulatory reforms are some of the challenges that will continue to impact the patient's healthcare experience.

Who the Book Is For and What the Book Covers

This book addresses how a strong nursing research agenda can impact patient care and influence the redesign of services needed to effectively respond to a changing healthcare environment. Nurse clinicians, leaders, administrators, educators, researchers, and students will find the information contained within this book informative and a valuable resource to guide the development of a research agenda in care delivery. Organizations interested in promoting a culture of inquiry will find examples from the MGH experience useful in explaining the importance of a nursing research agenda. Clinicians with a range of research expertise will hopefully find discussions about the support for and the conduct of research applicable to their professional and personal development. Doctorally prepared nurses will find examples of how to design a research infrastructure and the resources, support, and organizational commitment needed to promote research in practice settings. Clinicians, educators, and organizational leaders will hopefully find the content around mentoring, evidence-based practice, methods and evaluation, instrument development, and post-doctoral fellowships useful. Professional advances used to foster the development of new funding sources, partnerships, team-building, and engagement in multidisciplinary research activities are helpful, especially when explored in relationship to influencing organizational initiatives through nursing research and acquiring and sustaining Magnet® Recognition.

A book that is grounded in the philosophical and theoretical underpinnings of professional nursing can help guide the discovery of new knowledge and promote quality, evidenced-based, cost-effective care and link practice closely to research and care outcomes. This book seeks to accomplish this by also advancing goals within the *Institute of Medicine's Report on the Future of Nursing* (IOM; 2010) that address nursing leadership, the impact of nursing knowledge on healthcare reform and enhancement of safe, high-quality, cost-effective, patient/family-centric care through educational preparation and inquiry.

How This Book Is Organized

In this book's foreword, Angela McBride thoughtfully reflects, "I spent the major portion of my career in academia, largely because that was the arena where I saw the greatest opportunity for innovation and meaningful scholarship.... Now I'm not so sure that academe is the most dynamic place to be."

This book provides a comprehensive review to support the practice environment as an important place to advance nursing science through research. The introduction and remaining chapters help to articulate this insight by presenting essential elements needed to advance an active nursing research agenda within a multidisciplinary practice environment.

Chapter 1: Creating a Culture of Inquiry Within a Healthcare Medical Center

The current healthcare environment is ready for the integration of knowledge developed by nurse scholars for use in delivery of cost-effective, high-quality, efficient, safe patient-centric healthcare. This chapter expands the discussion of research within the framework of the Professional Practice Model at the Massachusetts General Hospital (Ives Erickson, Jones, & Ditomassi, 2013) and the development of a culture of inquiry to advance professional practice and improved patient care outcomes. The important role of nursing leadership and organizational commitment to research is presented along with the supports needed to foster a research infrastructure and enhance organizational excellence. Within this context, nurse scientists are in a position to develop a research trajectory that complements the organizational goals and address issues of importance to the health of the nation.

Chapter 2: Creating an Infrastructure that Enhances Professional Practice and Patient Care Services

This chapter focuses on the development, implementation, and expansion of the Institute for Patient Care (IPC) and the four centers that have been developed within the IPC. A brief discussion of each center will be provided. The chapter provides examples of how the work of the Yvonne L. Munn Center for Nursing Research interfaces with Patient Care Services and describes the synergistic relationship of the Munn Center with other centers within IPC and beyond (e.g., the MGH Research Institute).

Chapter 3: Promoting Nursing Research Through the Yvonne L. Munn Center

This chapter provides a comprehensive overview of the development and implementation of the Yvonne L. Munn Center for Nursing Research, including its mission, goals, team members, and role descriptions and infrastructure (e.g., meeting schedules, committee structure, policies, and grant development). The overall design of the center along with a discussion of the links to the Institute for Patient Care and Patient Care Services are expanded upon. Strategies used to promote a nursing research agenda within and across clinical settings are explored along with a description of efforts used to increase the visibility of research in staff, nurse scientists, external faculty nurse scientists, and other collaborators. Initiatives designed to promote inquiry (e.g. research awards, postdoctoral fellowships, doctoral forum, clinical nurse research task force) along with strategies to foster grant development and dissemination of research findings are discussed.

Chapter 4: Using, Evaluating, and Integrating an Evidence-Based Practice

The focus of this chapter is on differentiating terminology used around the development of original research, research utilization, performance improvement initiatives, and evidence-based practice (EBP). Exploration of an existing collaborative governance committee at the MGH to foster the development, use and translation of evidence is included. A discussion is also presented on strategies (e.g. grant funding) to foster staff engagement in evidence-driven practice. Examples of EBP projects are provided. Strategies to enhance the translation of evidence into practice are discussed along with evaluation of the EMR, documentation, standardized languages, and nursing research.

Chapter 5: Supporting Operational Effectiveness and Encouraging Research Through Innovation

This chapter focuses on the development, implementation, and evaluation of innovation across Patient Care Service (PCS) and includes staff and leadership involvement, strategic planning, project implementation, and program evaluation. Collaboration between and among nurse scientists and other disciplines is discussed and research evaluation strategies explored. The effectiveness of innovation will be discussed. Examples of innovations are presented along with a discussion of data collection, storage, and retrieval.

Chapter 6: Promoting Nursing Research in a Multidisciplinary Organization

This discussion elaborates of the collaborative approaches used to link nursing research activities to the larger organizational research enterprise (e.g. Partners Research Enterprise). Opportunities around nurse-led research initiatives, creating multidisciplinary research teams, and conducting research across disciplines are presented. Research resources at the organizational level will be discussed along with examples of educational programs offered support research development. Nursing membership on Institutional Review Boards and the development of research activities across the organization including nurse-led patient Advisory Committees and their influence on current funding mechanism (e.g. PCORI) will be explored.

Chapter 7: Research, Mentoring, and Developing Postdoctoral Scholars

This chapter explores the important role of mentoring for all nurses interested in research. National guidelines on the role of mentoring and nursing research will be presented and examples of mentoring practices discussed. Examples of funding, including philanthropic support and the development, implementation, and evaluation of the Connell Postdoctoral Nursing Research Scholars (CNRS) program and the role of mentorship in advancing scholars research will be presented. Opportunities to access internal and external funding and grant support within a clinical environment are provided.

Chapter 8: Evaluating Professional Practice in Nursing Research

An overview of the development and evaluation of the MGH professional practice model along with a discussion about measures used to evaluate its effectiveness. Specific areas of research concentration (e.g. ethics, workforce evaluation, disruptive behavior, staff satisfaction, leadership evaluation) are presented and methodologies used to advance the research. Examples of instruments developed within Patient Care Services and the Munn Center will be explored.

Chapter 9: The Magnet Recognition Program® Journey: An Engine for Research and Evidence-Based Practice

This chapter links the impact of nursing research and evidence-based practice examples to achieving and sustaining Magnet® recognition. The discussion focuses on the importance of healthcare environments developing and implementing a strong nursing research agenda to achieve the goals of within the Magnet Recognition Program® process. Examples that focus on the use of evidence and practice and policy changes that result will be presented.

Chapter 10: Concluding Thoughts

This final chapter will discuss the overall value and impact of an active nursing research agenda within the professional practice setting. Emphasis will be placed on the results of nursing inquiry and patient, family, and community outcomes. A discussion is provided to implement strategies needed to sustain and grow nursing and multidisciplinary research, advance research within the Munn Center and across PCS; including developing new partnerships, fostering multisite studies, expanding grant funding opportunities, generating new opportunism for mentoring nurse researchers, and extending nursing research to a global community of nurse scholars. Concluding thoughts on the future of nursing research in healthcare will be provided along with the added contribution of nursing's unique perspective on the patient experiences informing the challenges of healthcare reform.

References

Institute of Medicine (IOM) (2010). *The future of nursing: Leading the change, advancing health.* Washington, DC: The National Academies Press.

Ives Erickson, J., Jones, D., Ditomassi, M. (2013). *Fostering nurse-led care.* Indianapolis, IN: Sigma Theta Tau International.

Chapter 1

Creating a Culture of Inquiry Within a Healthcare Medical Center

–Jeanette Ives Erickson, DNP, RN, NEA-BC, FAAN

Florence Nightingale, the founder of modern-day nursing, ensured that nursing research was an integral component of her agenda for change. Nightingale identified relevant issues impacting the morbidity and mortality of soldiers during the Crimean War. Her hypothesis, development, collection of data, and systematic review of literature led her to find solutions to vexing problems that had gone unsolved and treated. Her work resulted in changes in practice and within the environment of care. Her research was holistic in that she integrated nursing with all facets of society (Dossey, 2005, p. 122). Today, we view her work as the development and application of evidence-based practice (EBP).

In the 21st century, nursing continues to address healthcare challenges, including globalization, which drives the necessity to have a clear focus on healthcare delivery, to apply current knowledge and methods, and to develop new knowledge to transform the future of nursing. The current healthcare environment is ripe for the integration of nursing knowledge developed by nurse scholars for the delivery of cost-effective, high-quality, efficient, safe, timely, equitable, patient-centric healthcare (Institute of Medicine [IOM], 2001). Visionary leadership, along with the increased presence of doctorally prepared nurses in clinical practice, has created a unique environment to develop, test, refine, and extend knowledge at the bedside for patients and families in the hospital, as well as in the communities and in health centers.

This chapter discusses the importance of creating an agenda for change through advancing a culture of inquiry in an organization that values nursing knowledge and the unique contributions of nurses to patient care and to the interdisciplinary team. The author utilizes personal experience as a chief nurse within a major academic medical center where research historically was primarily dominated by medicine to introduce nursing research as another important way to improve care. The value of articulating the impact of nursing knowledge on the organization is showcased within this chapter in two ways:

- The journey to develop a robust nursing research agenda

- The creation of a center for nursing research

The sections that follow address these real-life experiences.

Creating the Agenda for Change

Throughout her distinguished career, Yvonne, L. Munn, RN, chief nurse at Boston's Massachusetts General Hospital from 1984 to 1993, promoted evidence-based, patient-focused practice within a primary nursing model of care. Her vision was that through inquiry and lifelong learning nurses could articulate and solve important problems impacting patients and organizational effectiveness. Upon Mrs. Munn's retirement, her executive team honored her by making personal financial contributions toward the launch of the annual Yvonne L. Munn Research Lecture. Peter Beurhaus, a nurse and healthcare economist, was the inaugural Munn lecturer in 1993. (See Table 1.1 for a listing of all presenters.)

TABLE 1.1 Annual Yvonne L. Munn Nursing Research Lecturers

YEAR	YLM NURSING RESEARCH LECTURER	PRESENTATION TITLE
2014	Elizabeth Ann Manhart Barrett, PhD, RN-BC, LHMC, FAAN	Implementing Power as Knowing Participation in Change: Impact on the Professional Practice Environment
2013	Susan Moorhead, PhD, RN, FAAN	Communicating Nursing's Impact on Patient Outcomes Through the Use of Standardized Nursing Terminologies
2012	Jeffrey M. Adams, PhD, RN	The Bucket List: Advancing an International Research Agenda Using Administrative Data in the Evaluation of Leadership and Organizations
2011	Laurie M. Lauzon Clabo, PhD, RN	Patient Care Units as Cultures of Practice: The Way We Do Things Here
2010	Susan Gennaro, DSN, RN, FAAN	From the NICU to OB Clinics: A Research Journey
2009	Linda Aiken, PhD, RN, FAAN, FRCN	Pursuit of Quality
2008	Nancy S. Redeker, PhD, RN, FAHA, FAAN	Sleep Deprivation in Acute Care: Priority or Afterthought
2007	Cheryl Tatano Beck, DNSc, CNM, FAAN	Cultivating a Program of Research: Merging Clinical and Research Interests
2006	Loretta Sweet Jemmott, PhD, RN, FAAN	The Nurse Scientist: Blazing New Trails in Health Promotion
2005	Ruth McCorkle, PhD, RN, FAAN	From the Bedside to Research and Back Again
2004	Lorraine Mion, PhD, RN, FAAN	Care of the Elderly: Making a Difference through Research
2003	Margaret Grey, RN, DrPH, FAAN	Enhancing Behavioral Care for Youths with Diabetes

continues

TABLE 1.1 *continued*

YEAR	YLM NURSING RESEARCH LECTURER	PRESENTATION TITLE
2002	Barbara Wolfe, PhD, RN, PMHCNS-BC, FAAN	Nursing Research: Improving Patient Care through Clinical Inquiry
2001	Terry Fulmer, PhD, RN, FAAN	Nurses Improving Care of the Health Services Elderly (NICHE)
2000	JoEllen W. Hawkins, PhD, RNC, FAAN	Research: From the Ivory Tower to the Bedside
1999	Lin Zhan, PhD, RN, FAAN	Asian American Voices: Asian and Asian-American Health Educators Speak Out
1998	Dorothy A. Jones, EdD, RN, FAAN, FNI	Creating a Climate for Research-Based Practice
1997	Martha A. Curley, PhD, RN, FAAN	Nursing's Unique Contribution to Patient Outcomes
1996	Dolores Krieger, PhD, RN	Creative Clinical Aspects of Therapeutic Touch
1995	Sara T. Fry, PhD, RN, FAAN	Must Health Professionals Always Tell the Patient the Truth?
1993	Peter I. Beurhaus, PhD, RN, FAAN	Health Care Reform and Critical Issues Confronting Nurses

Held annually during Nurse Recognition Week, the Munn Nursing Research Lecture, a component of Nursing Research Day, hosts nurse researchers from around the world. The day provides opportunities to share new information and to challenge nurses and others "to identify new ways to shape and influence nursing practice" (The Yvonne L. Munn Center for Nursing Research, 2008, p. 14). The yearly invitational Munn Nursing Research Lecture was step one of the journey to develop a robust nursing research agenda. But as the new chief nurse, the author understood that this was not enough to create a culture change whereby nursing knowledge, inquiry, and research would be viewed as making a difference and the contributions impacting healthcare. Thus, the Yvonne L. Munn Center for Nursing Research emerged over time (as discussed in detail in Chapter 2, "Creating an Infrastructure that Enhances Professional Practice and Patient Care Services," and Chapter 3, "Promoting Nursing Research Through the Yvonne L. Munn Center"). The Munn Center created new visibility for nursing and its impact on care, developing and using evidence and creating opportunities for all nurses to participate in the evolution of research through mentoring and partnering with others to advance patient care.

Integrating Nursing Inquiry into the Philosophy of Care Delivery

To develop a culture of inquiry, it was important to define a strategy that embedded nursing knowledge into clinical practice. This required creating a framework to align all stakeholders across the inter-professional team guiding professional practice. It also required the core infrastructure necessary to "explore, develop, learn and articulate" each discipline's contributions to patient care (Ives Erickson, 2013, p. 7) to the organization and to the profession. At Massachusetts General Hospital (MGH), we articulated this framework in the form of a Professional Practice Model (PPM (Ives Erickson, 2013)). The model is grounded in the organization's mission, vision, values, and guiding principles. The guiding principles clearly articulate a commitment to knowledge generation, including the following (Jones & Kacmarek, 2007, pp. 12–13):

- Creating a practice environment that fosters a spirit of inquiry
- Developing new knowledge and testing that knowledge within the clinical practice environment
- Translating knowledge into practice to impact patient-care outcomes and the overall patient experience
- Generating and using evidence to inform practice and improve outcomes

Figure 1.1 demonstrates the importance of research and EBP as part of the important framework advancing practice. As one of nine interlocking pieces comprising the key components in a strong professional practice environment, which are shown in the following list, research and EBP play an important role:

- Research and evidence-based practice (EBP)

- Vision and values

- Standards of practice

- Narrative culture

- Professional development and lifelong learning

- Relationship-based care

- Clinical recognition and advancement

- Collaborative decision-making

- Innovation and entrepreneurial teamwork

Research and EBP are an integral part of every nurse's role. Chapter 8, "Evaluating Professional Practice in Nursing Research," discusses this model and its impact on staff satisfaction within the professional practice environment in detail.

Alignment through a PPM is core to the evolution of a culture change. In addition, the PPM helped set the stage for a major research agenda was set with the development of Nursing Research Day. But these two initiatives (Nursing Research Day and the launch of the Yvonne L. Munn Center for Nursing Research) were only the beginning of the agenda for change at this major academic medical center. It was the belief of the chief nurse and the nursing executive team that the care provided by the clinical nursing staff must be built upon a foundation of knowledge and a spirit of inquiry and discovery, with a goal of generating research that would advance high-quality, safe care. According to Moule and Goodman (2009), nurses need to be research-aware and require the skills identified in the following list:

- Capacity for critical thinking

- Analytical skills

- Skills to gain access to relevant research evidence

- Critical understanding of research processes

- Ability to read and critically appraise research and other types of evidence

- An awareness of ethical issues related to research

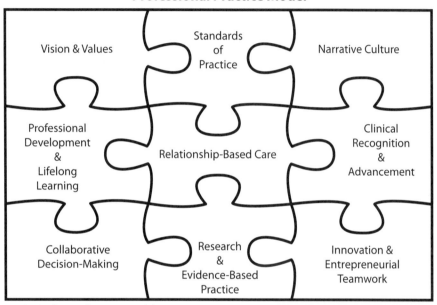

© MGH Professional Practice Model, 2014

FIGURE 1.1

MGH Professional Practice Model

Creating a Learning Environment

For nurses to develop research skills and expertise in the conduct of research, the chief nurse has a responsibility to create learning opportunities, to identify mentors and other resources for nurses to keep up to date on emerging best practices, to use research and evidence in the development of the patients plan of care, and to provide opportunities to unbundle unique patient problems and discover new ways to care for patients.

It is easy for a chief nurse to get caught up in the day-to-day issues of shortages within the workforce, hospital overcrowding, and constraints within the fiscal environment. However, creating this agenda for change does not necessarily require the acquisition of new full-time employees (FTEs). The more important resource a chief nurse has is the coalition of willing nurses. In most organizations, nurses in almost every specialty area participate in journal clubs, further their education, precept new nurses and nursing students, attend professional development programs, become certified in a clinical specialty, and/or read the literature. The chief nurse has a responsibility and opportunity to seize upon this core value of nurses to continuously self-improve, to participate in new ways to advance their care team, and to improve the care they and their colleagues deliver to the patients they serve.

For any organization, the presence of nursing faculty within the practice environment can become a core opportunity for research training and the advancement of scholarly work. Partnerships created through the alignment with faculty having nurse scientist appointments help faculty advance their program of research and offer cost-effective ways to advance a research agenda. This includes:

- Promoting a program of research

- Including faculty in clinical staff research programs

- Serving as mentors to facilitate inquiry

- Participation on grant reviews, abstract reviews, and working toward joint publications

There are numerous and creative mechanisms for mutual benefit that advance the impact of nursing research in clinical and administrative practice. Chapter 3 provides a more complete discussion of these activities.

Extending Research Beyond the Medical Staff

The politics of research is interesting in that some believe nurses do not conduct or utilize research. Though the growth of nursing research has been slow, early nurse researchers such as Dorothy A. Jones, a faculty member at an area college of nursing, understood that nurse leaders and educators had a responsibility to disseminate EBP and to embed research into core nursing curriculums. This was key to fostering research at a school of nursing, which was also grounded in an appointment in an academic medical center as a nurse scientist. Jones is not unique in this action, but her ability to align with the chief nurse and others, taking core concepts and belief systems and putting them into a plan, is indeed unique and has proven invaluable. Jones's ability to bridge service and academics allowed us to launch a broad-scale research agenda to design, develop, and launch a center for nursing research. Jones's work launching the Yvonne L. Munn Center for Nursing Research is discussed in depth in Chapter 3.

Concurrently, Marianne Ditomassi, Director of Education at the time, focused on developing the Center for Clinical and Professional Development. The vision for the center was to embrace the importance of continuing education and the creation of opportunities to advance each nurse's professional career through lifelong learning. A robust certification program, residencies, and a professional advancement program emerged grounded in the teachings of Patricia Benner. Utilizing the Dreyfus Model of Skill Acquisition (Dreyfus & Dreyfus, 1986), Benner published *From Novice to Expert: Excellence and Power in Clinical Practice* (1984), which articulated how nurses develop clinical knowledge through experience, formal education, and reflection. Benner's work, described in the narratives of practicing nurses, reported the evolving stages from novice practice to expert practice. In novice practice, there is a reliance on rules, a situation is made up of equally relevant parts, and the focus is less on the task than the patient. In expert practice, there is less reliance on rules than on past experience, the most salient aspects of a situation are relevant, and the nurse is fully engaged and involved with the patient and family.

The chief nurse understood the need for synergy between education, professional advancement, and an opportunity to change practice and to discover new ways of doing and knowing. The development of work within the nursing service was designed to ensure that once the strategic plan was developed, the strategies could be disseminated and the tactics implemented.

As the strategic and operational plan was being designed, the chief nurse began to enlist key stakeholders within the organization, including physician colleagues, the CEO, members of the administration, and an important ally, the development office. In 1996, when this plan was being developed, healthcare organizations were addressing the rising costs of healthcare, and consultants were advising organizations to develop new nursing staffing models that replaced registered nurses (RNs) with unlicensed assistive personnel to perform tasks that did not require RN licensure but rather a delegation by the RN to others. The message was clear: There were no discretionary funds to launch a nursing research program. It was the belief of the chief nurse and her executive team that while the economic factors were powerful, the organization would be more powerful working as a whole. By building a coalition of believers, the plan to launch the two new centers (the Yvonne L. Munn Center for Nursing Research and the Center for Clinical and Professional Development) was put into place. Physician and administrative colleagues understood that the core mission of the organization of patient care, education, and research was a shared mission and not reserved for the medical staff alone.

Promoting a Research Agenda for Nurses: The Role of the CNO

One of the early multisite nursing research studies was the Magnet® Hospital Study (McClure, Poulin, Sovie, & Wandelt, 1983) chartered by the American Academy of Nursing (AAN) to identify work environments that attracted and retained nurses who provide high-quality patient care. Only 41 of 163 healthcare organizations studied were identified as having the qualities needed to create an environment that empowered nurses. Today, only 7% (401 of 5,686) of hospitals in the United States and 8 international hospitals are Magnet-recognized. In 2008, the Commission on Magnet Recognition created a new conceptual model that identified key components thought to embody a new vision for Magnet-recognized hospitals (ANCC, 2008):

- ANCC Magnet-recognized organizations will serve as the fount of knowledge and expertise for the delivery of nursing care globally.

- They will be solidly grounded in core Magnet principles, flexible, and constantly striving for discovery and innovation.

- They will lead the reformation of healthcare; the discipline of nursing; and care of the patient, family, and community.

Chapter 9, "The Magnet Recognition Program® Journey: An Engine for Research and Evidence-Based Practice," discusses the components and Magnet program and its impact in advancing the nursing research agenda at length.

The Magnet® Model is important when a chief nursing officer (CNO) considers the development of a nursing research program and/or center for nursing research, because the focus on the support, conduct, and application of research to clinical and administrative practice is helpful. The CNO, as a visionary nurse and organizational leader, needs to demonstrate the ability to advance a research agenda, especially within a clinical practice environment. The CNO must be able to link research to an organizational mission, along with aligning with national research agendas. Many chief nurses today are seasoned scholars with a wide range of experiences, including organizational leadership and mentors of selected graduate nursing students (including dissertations, research projects, grant reviewer). In addition, they are also well-published scholars, having presented in both national and international forums. The CNO is an advisor and mentor to emerging leaders, assisting scholars with the development of a research plan. The link to the Magnet Recognition Program® work helped to solidify the chief nurse's committment to the development of a Nursing Research Center.

Articulating the Focus

Decisions about the focus of nursing research evolve over time, but those decisions must also align with the needs of the staff and the patients served. Our patient population spans the spectrum of life from birth to death. Therefore, the first aspect of the focus for embedding discovery into practice was to focus on EBP. Developing areas of research foci emerged in concert with the strategic goals of the organization. They included the following:

- Care of the elderly

- Ethics and decision-making

- Symptom management, including pressure ulcers, pain, and risk for injury (e.g., patient falls)

- Workforce evaluation

- Health services research

- Complementary healing interventions

- The articulation of problem solving and process dialogue to impact care

In addition, advancing programs of research through internal and external funding modalities helped expand clinical investigation and resulted in outcomes to support the impact of new ideas on care. Use of multiple methodologies, including quantitative and qualitative research (along with the development of a battery of instruments and an expanded website), has extended the impact of the Munn Center and increased the visibility of its contributions nationally and beyond. Throughout this book, multiple chapters address aspects of the implementation of a nursing research agenda, providing greater detail to help guide others as they advance a nursing research agenda within a clinical practice site.

Understanding the Lessons Learned

From the vantage point of a chief nurse advancing the research agenda for years, the author has learned several lessons.

- Start small. Identify a first step on your research journey (e.g., journal club, launch an EBP committee, provide mini-grants to support conduct of research).

- Adopt a long-term time horizon. It takes time to "seed" a culture of inquiry.

- Make research visible. Seize every opportunity to showcase nursing research outcomes or application of research.

- Build the bench strength of resources to provide support and mentorship. Cultivate a network of researchers within and outside the walls of the organization.

- Create the infrastructure to support research operations.

- Develop a coalition of investors through fundraising and grant writing.

Summary

An emerging focus on care is the evaluation of patient outcomes and the impact of nurse-driven care interventions on care indicators and outcomes, including cost, length of stay, and rehospitalizations and emergency department visits. This chapter begins to link the development of a research agenda to advance care strategies and to unbundle knowledge embedded in innovative delivery models. Critical to future research will be the creation of a culture that values the development and use of evidence to guide practice, the translation of research findings to impact direct care, research collaborations and partnerships with other disciplines, and the patients and families in broad clinical investigations who will create knowledge needed to address the challenges of healthcare by nurses and other providers.

Equally important is the emphasis a healthcare organization places on the evaluation of efforts that promote patient and family satisfaction and strategies that promote a care environment to enhance nursing's ability to integrate knowledge into practice. In addition, all of the following depend on clinical investigations that foster nursing knowledge, collaboration, and strategies that impact health outcomes and reduce costs:

- Evaluation of innovation technology and optimization of staff's commitment to improve the health of society

- Better understanding of the patient/family healthcare experience

- Introducing research-based strategies to promote health, foster spiritual well-being, promote reflection and healing, improve illness management, and reduce suffering

The activities of nurse researchers at the MGH complement the research agendas of patient care services as well as the organization and external funding agencies, including Health Services Research Agency, the National Institutes of Health, and the National Institute of Nursing Research. In addition, these initiatives also speak to the goals of the Institute of Medicine report on *The Future of Nursing: Leading Change, Advancing Health* (2010). To encourage nurses to practice at the top of their profession, the nurse researchers at the MGH have begun a concerted effort to address topics of importance to the health of the nation and beyond. Research activities span diverse populations, including the underserved, culturally diverse, and vulnerable, in addition to those settings that offer new opportunities (e.g., the home, rehabilitation centers, and nursing homes) for managing patients and supporting families outside of the acute care environment.

Today, the Yvonne L. Munn Center for Nursing Research at MGH is a highly respected and valued nursing research program, but but it takes time and dedication to grow. The Munn Center has achieved international visibility for advancing clinical research and development of nurse scientist and postdoctoral scholars within the United States and abroad. It has designed and developed scholars within the Munn Center, and has also linked with nurses throughout the MGH to advance clinical scholarship through engagement in science and dissemination of their work through global presentations and publications. This community of scholars includes clinical nurses, advanced practice registered nurses, doctorally prepared nurses, and nurse partners from other clinical sites as well as academic institutions from multiple sites, nationally and internationally. It is more than a space; it is a value and an ideal. Nursing practice at the MGH is evidence-based and research-driven. The journey and resulting culture change required organizational commitment and agreement that nursing research needed to be a major component in the very fabric of the organization. Through this work, we bring new knowledge to interdisciplinary research teams seeking to improve patient care.

References

American Nurses Credentialing Center (ANCC). (2008). *A New Model for ANCC's Magnet Recognition Program®*. Silver Spring, MD: American Nurses Credentialing Center.

Benner, P. (1984). *From novice to expert: Excellence and power in clinical nursing practice.* Menlo Park, CA: Addison-Wesley Publishing Company.

Dossey, B. M. (2006). Florence Nightingale: The passionate statistician. In B. M. Dossey, L. C. Selanders, D. Beck, & A. Attewell. (Eds), *Florence Nightingale today: Healing, leadership & global action.* Silver Spring, MD: American Nurses Association.

Dreyfus, H. L., & Dreyfus, S. E. (1986). *Mind over machine: The power of human intuition and expertise in the era of the computer.* New York: The Free Press.

Institute of Medicine (IOM). (2001). *Crossing the quality chasm: A new health system for the 21st century,* Washington, DC: The National Academy Press.

Institute of Medicine (IOM). (2010). *The future of nursing: Leading change, advancing health.* Washington, DC: The National Academy Press.

Ives Erickson, J. (2013). Influencing professional practice at the bedside. In J. Ives Erickson, D. A. Jones, & M. Ditomassi (Eds). *Fostering nurse-led care: Professional practice for the bedside leader from Massachusetts General Hospital.* Indianapolis, IN: Sigma Theta Tau.

Jones, D. A., & Kacmarek, R. (2007). Research: Fostering a spirit of inquiry of patient care. *Caring Headlines,* April 5, 2007.

McClure, M., Poulin, M., Sovie, M., & Wandelt, M. (1983). *Magnet® Hospitals: Attraction and Retention of Professional Nurses.* American Academy of Nursing Task Force on Nursing Practice in Hospitals. Kansas City, MO: American Nurses Association.

Moule, P., & Goodman, M. (2009). *Nursing research: An introduction.* London, England: Sage.

The Yvonne L. Munn Center for Nursing Research. (2008). Nursing research opportunities abound. *Caring Headlines,* November 20, 2008.

Chapter 2
Creating an Infrastructure that Enhances Professional Practice and Patient Care Services

–*Gaurdia Banister, PhD, RN, FAAN*

The current healthcare environment continues to seek new ways to respond to the complex challenges of healthcare delivery for patients and their families. Pressures directed at enhancing evidence-based practice (EBP), culturally responsive and patient-centric care, and integration of initiatives to reduce cost, improve quality and safety, and effectively measure and monitor change and sustainability of innovation require a new vision, expertise, and resources.

The Institute of Medicine's (IOM) reports and significant publications in recent years (e.g., *Crossing the Quality Chasm* [2001], *Unequal Treatment: Confronting Racial and Ethnic Disparities in Healthcare* [2003], *The Future of Nursing: Leading Change, Advancing Health* [2010], and *Integrating Research and Practice: Health System Leaders Working Toward High-Value Care: Workshop Summary* [2014]) have all highlighted the need for changes in healthcare delivery. These changes include the generation of new care delivery models and structures needed to increase efficiencies, produce new knowledge, and promote incorporation of new learning competencies. One structure that can guide these developments is a well-designed, fully implemented Professional Practice

Model (PPM) that can integrate an emerging vision and provide needed resources and expertise required to support inquiry and enhance development, implementation, and evaluation of care redesign.

The mission of the Massachusetts General Hospital (MGH) (2009) offers a commitment to excellence in the delivery of care:

> *"Guided by the needs of our patients and their families, we aim to deliver the very best healthcare in a safe, compassionate environment; to advance that care through innovative research and education; and, to improve the health and well-being of the diverse communities we serve."*

Honoring the commitment to achieving this mission has guided the leadership of the senior vice president for patient care and chief nurse in creating and sustaining a professional practice environment that works each day to actualize this mission in all aspects of patient- and family-centered care.

The PPM (Ives Erickson, Ditomassi, & Jones, 2013), as discussed in Chapter 1, "Creating a Culture of Inquiry Within a Healthcare Medical Center," and Chapter 8, "Evaluating Professional Practice in Nursing Research," was introduced by the chief nurse in 1996. The PPM has served as a framework to guide the work of nurses and other disciplines within patient care services (PCS). The model works to build on the salient elements of autonomy, control over practice, and collaborative relationships with physicians (Ives Erickson & Ditomassi, 2012) to optimize a multidisciplinary approach that enhances all dimensions of care. The patient and family are central to the implementation of this model, providing relationship-based care within the scope and responsibility of a discipline's professional scope of practice. Building on that foundation, the constructs of this PPM reflect the ideas of staff committees and interdisciplinary teams empowered to bring voice to their practice. The following list describes the elements of this model (Ives Erickson, Ditomassi & Jones, 2008):

- Promotion of relationship-based care

- A clinical practice that is anchored by our vision and values and defined by standards

- Promotion of innovation and interprofessional teamwork

- A commitment to collaborative decision-making where the accountability and authority for practice resides in the clinicians

- Clinical and professional development aimed at lifelong learning

- Awards, staff recognition, and professional advancement

- Embedding a narrative culture to foster promotion of experiential learning

- Developing and advancing evidence-based practice

The Institute for Patient Care

"We're bringing together our work in patient care, education and research to plan for the next year, the next decade and the legacy we want to leave into the next century." –Jeanette Ives Erickson, 2006

The Institute for Patient Care (IPC) was created in 2007 to embody and support the elements of the PPM. The IPC is a dynamic constellation of centers and programmatic initiatives that serve to actualize professional practice within Patient Care Services (PCS) and enhance patient- and family-centered care. The IPC is a key component of PCS and is involved in promoting the education and professional development of staff, supporting and recognizing clinical advancement, generating new knowledge, and creating opportunities to participate actively in collaborative decision-making across disciplines. Centers within the IPC are engaged in promoting and evaluating the impact of innovation; celebrating discovery and sharing knowledge; and developing, using, and evaluating evidence-based care to optimize care at the bedside.

The overarching goal of the IPC is to promote synergy and collaboration across the centers to advance interdisciplinary clinical work within PCS. The institute provides nurses, therapists, social workers, and other PCS staff with opportunities for development and personal growth by providing new knowledge and experiences needed to advance professional goals and enhance patient and family care. The values and beliefs of PCS are embodied in and exemplified by professional strategies that promote education, research, and innovation.

Institute priorities are set by the PCS executive team. The leaders across the centers, along with the executive director, have the flexibility and adaptability needed to address emerging priorities and unanticipated needs, including new staffing requirements, development of programs for staff that respond to the demands of changing regulations, improving quality and safety, survey results, or organizational mandates. The current goals of the institute (as revised in 2012) are actualized and embedded into the organizational culture for long-term sustainability and are as follows:

- Foster an environment of clinical inquiry and experiential learning.

- Create a synergy across all centers and programmatic initiatives to advance the goals of IPC.

- Work collaboratively to promote interdisciplinary team learning to optimize safe, effective patient care.

- Participate in the development and evaluation of organizational initiatives and individual and group programs of research.

- Seek multiple funding opportunities to advance the work of the institute and centers.

- Create opportunities to be present in the organization at the point of care and within committees across the organization.

- Assume leadership for innovation in evidence-based clinical practice.

- Support research that advances safe and effective evidence-based care.

- Provide leadership for innovations for staff, patients, and families in learning.

- Develop, implement, and evaluate programmatic initiatives that impact staff and patient outcomes.

- Advance the PCS's agenda to foster interdisciplinary practice to advance patient care.

- Disseminate the work of the institute and related centers through multiple local, national, and international forms.

Implementing the Goals of the IPC

The institute advances nursing and interdisciplinary practice through programs and initiatives, including collaborative governance, the clinical recognition program, clinical simulation, and other awards and recognition programs. The institute works to encourage efficient use of resources, to promote learning, and to research initiatives that can be developed and supported by internal and external funding sources. The ongoing development of learning resources for staff, patients, and families focuses on the promotion of culturally sensitive, safe, and effective patient care.

The institute assumes a leadership role in creating new directions for professional development and advancement through increased mentoring opportunities. The IPC and centers collaborate with a number of constituents, including the PCS executive team, nursing directors, clinical nurse specialists, clinical nurses, and interdisciplinary staff, in addition to physicians, students, faculty, patients, and families. The staff works through and with clinicians and care team members who are critical to care delivery. For example, clinical nurse specialists (CNSs) working in the IPC use their expertise in quality patient care by focusing on indicators such as pressure ulcers, pain, geriatrics, and ethics to lead evidence-based initiatives that impact staff and patients. They lead major initiatives such as the pressure ulcer task force, the pain management project, and ethics and decision-making forums to consult with staff and patients to improve outcomes. The CNSs working in the IPC, whom are doctorally prepared nurses, generate and advance knowledge through research and implement quality-improvement projects within their specialized practice area.

Multidisciplinary projects designed to complement and enhance patient care and professional development are encouraged and supported. These projects include the interprofessional dedicated education unit that focuses on the development of competencies for team based education and clinical practice. The disciplines of nursing, speech language pathology and physical therapy are involved in this innovative initiative. Our simulation programs, many of which are multidisciplinary such as code team training and caring for patients with acute changes in mental status, embrace the themes of leadership, communication, teamwork, decision-making, and application of clinical knowledge as disciplines collaborate to provide new knowledge.

The Centers Within the Institute

Within the IPC, four centers work collaboratively to achieve the goals of the institute:

- The Norman Knight Nursing Center for Clinical & Professional Development
- The Maxwell & Eleanor Blum Patient & Family Learning Center
- The Yvonne L. Munn Center for Nursing Research
- The Center for Innovations in Care Delivery

Each center has a strategic role within the institute and is fundamental to achieving and exceeding the goals of PCS. Figure 2.1 provides an overview of the mission and objectives of the IPC and its four centers.

The Norman Knight Center for Clinical & Professional Development

Established in 1997, the Norman Knight Nursing Center for Clinical & Professional Development focuses on the dissemination and utilization of knowledge for the attainment of safe, effective, and competent patient- and family-centered nursing practice. The center staff work to accomplish this goal through several product lines, including orientation and onboarding, new course development, eLearning and management of the learning management system, educational project management, educational consultation, in-service training, and serving as an American Nurses Credentialing Center-approved provider unit for continuing nursing education. Underscoring these services is its mission:

> "To promote lifelong learning and clinical excellence by establishing, supporting and fostering learning opportunities for the attainment of knowledge and skills necessary for safe, competent and compassionate patient-centered care."

THE INSTITUTE FOR PATIENT CARE

ADVANCING ORGANIZATIONAL INTERDISCIPLINARY INITIATIVES

The Institute for Patient Care (IPC) consists of a collaborative of centers, programs, and initiatives designed to lead and support excellence in interdisciplinary clinical work in Patient Care Services and throughout the MGH.

The mission of the IPC is to support and create new directions for professional development, to ensure that patients and families are educated consumers of care, and to generate, disseminate, and integrate research in delivering evidence-based practice with the ultimate goal of providing safe, timely, efficient, cost-effective, and high-quality care.

Initiatives include:
- Awards and Recognition Program
- Clinical Affiliations
- Clinical Recognition Program
- Collaborative Governance
- Consultation
- Credentialing
- Ethical and Clinical Decision-making

- Global Nursing Education
- Leadership Development
- Organizational Evaluation
- Organizational Patient Care Initiatives, e.g., falls, geriatrics, pressure ulcers, pain relief
- Simulation Education
- Workforce Development

THE NORMAN KNIGHT NURSING CENTER FOR CLINICAL & PROFESSIONAL DEVELOPMENT	**THE YVONNE L. MUNN CENTER FOR NURSING RESEARCH**
Focus is on the dissemination and utilization of knowledge for the attainment of safe, effective, & competent patient & family-centered nursing practice.	Focus is on the development and utilization of nursing knowledge to improve patient care and optimize professional nursing practice.
THE MAXWELL & ELEANOR BLUM PATIENT & FAMILY LEARNING CENTER	**THE CENTER FOR INNOVATIONS IN CARE DELIVERY**
Focus is on providing the highest quality patient education and consumer health information services to MGH patients, families, and staff.	Focus is on bringing teams together to identify opportunities, estimate the impact of change, and construct innovations.

http://www.mghpcs.org/IPC/

FIGURE 2.1

IPC Goals and Center Objectives

The mission is the cornerstone of the Norman Knight Nursing Center and is brought to life through its programming. The multiple programs offered by the Knight Center are responsive to a learning needs survey conducted every 24–30 months, informed by the goals of PCS and provide learning opportunities that address learning needs of nurses at various experiential levels. Using a model of progressive mastery, the curriculums borrow from Benner's (1984) Novice to Expert framework and Senge's (1990) conceptual framework of a learning environment.

The Maxwell & Eleanor Blum Patient & Family Learning Center

The Maxwell & Eleanor Blum Patient & Family Learning Center is a state-of-the-art consumer health education resource center whose mission is to provide the highest quality patient and family education and health information services to the diverse community of MGH patients, families, and staff. It was established in 1999 and is now visited by an average of 24,000 people annually.

The vision of the Blum Center is to make patient education and consumer health information services accessible to all patients, families, employees, and staff of MGH through partnerships with the community, use of state-of-the-art technology, and access to comprehensive patient education services. The goals of the Blum Center include the following:

- Enabling patients and their families to learn about their health, illness, and healthcare through independent and assisted research

- Supporting health literacy by providing a structure for the development, dissemination, review, and approval of MGH patient education materials

- Assisting staff in acquiring the skills necessary to learn for themselves and effectively teach patients about health and illness.

Although the overarching goals of the center have remained the same, the focus of the work of the Blum Center has expanded primarily in the area of health literacy. Staff are embedded in care redesign teams where issues of patient education—content and process—are discussed at the advent, thus ensuring that as our approach to care changes so does our approach to patient education.

The Center for Innovations in Care Delivery

The Center for Innovations in Care Delivery, established in 2006, seeks to encourage creative, multidisciplinary practice within PCS. The center is designed to accelerate innovation; foster collaboration; and identify, prepare, and lead in creating a new vision of healthcare for the future. The center emphasizes the development, advancement, and interrelated nature of those initiatives that stimulate innovative products and processes. Toward this end, the center openly engages the MGH workforce, patients, and external organizations to engage in dialogue within a team-based approach to generate new ideas and engage in creative approaches to solve problems. The Center for Innovation in Care Delivery draws on the knowledge of multiple disciplines within the PCS workforce and embraces national and international collaborators in seeking visionary ways to address care delivery issues.

This center also works closely with the Yvonne L. Munn Center for Nursing Research to promote research opportunities and develop evaluation strategies related to the impact of changes within patient care and the workforce. Chapter 6, "Promoting Nursing Research in a Multidisciplinary Organization," provides a more complete discussion about the Center for Innovations in Care Delivery and its outcomes.

The Yvonne L. Munn Center for Nursing Research

Nursing research and the promotion of EBP, are essential components of the PPM and are realized through the efforts of this center's and programmatic initiatives of the institute. The Yvonne L. Munn Center for Nursing Research (Munn Center) opened in 2007, offering nurses at the MGH an opportunity to generate, translate, use, and disseminate nursing research to improve patient care. The Munn Center focuses on the utilization of existing research and the development, testing, evaluation, and refinement of new knowledge to inform practice decisions and improve the care of patients and families. As nurses engage in the research process, they become active participants in the discovery of knowledge needed to advance patient care and improve patient outcomes.

Opportunities to engage in nursing research exist across settings and populations and within all dimensions of professional nursing. The Munn Center provides an infrastructure to generate and mobilize resources and support nursing research initiatives related to PCS goals and strategic initiatives and advance clinical practice. Collaboration with staff in the Munn Center can result in the development of internal and external grants that support research initiatives and stimulate discovery. Findings from research investigations are presented to the MGH community at large and disseminated in the literature. The Munn Center supports an environment of inquiry that promotes discovery and generates knowledge needed to improve quality patient care outcomes and to facilitate collaboration across the centers within the institute and with other disciplines. Chapter 3, "Promoting Nursing Research Through the Yvonne L. Munn Center," provides an in-depth discussion of the overall structure and outcomes linked to the work of the Munn Center.

Outcomes of the Institute

Since the creation of the Institute for Patient Care, measurable outcomes have been achieved that reflect its impact and influence on the practice environment. Positioning the four centers and programmatic initiatives under one organizational structure has promoted collaboration, generated synergies, and created new and vital linkages that have impacted the patient care environment. The following subsections highlight a number of exemplars and outcomes to demonstrate the work of IPC in advancing knowledge development, innovating care delivery, advancing diversity, and promoting inquiry.

Knowledge Development

Goal: To strengthen the knowledge base of nurses to advance critical decision-making and promote skill acquisition

Outcome/exemplar: Critical-care nurse residency; preparing the next generation of nurses

The challenge: The impetus for the program emerged from the rising volume of patients requiring critical care, the opening of a new ICU, increasing clinical demands on staff, and a forecasted nursing shortage. This "perfect storm" challenged leadership to develop new approaches to the recruitment and retention of critical-care nurses, including an untapped pool of newly graduated nurses.

The response: The Norman Knight Nursing Center for Clinical & Professional Development created an innovative model to orient 50 newly graduated nurses (residents) to critical-care practice; the average number of residents was generally eight per critical-care unit/practice area. A small group of nurse-partners (preceptors) were assigned to each resident because of variations in work schedules. In addition to clinical orientation at the bedside, the residents received additional exposure to course content through lectures, clinical simulation scenarios, and skills practice sessions. Over time, the course content was expanded in selected areas such as electrolyte imbalances, ethics, and death and dying in response to residents' feedback on summative evaluations.

Evaluation: To evaluate its effectiveness, 12 focus groups were held to obtain input from each group involved in the program, including newly graduated nurse residents, nurse partners/preceptors, clinical nurse specialists, and nurse directors. Two independent reviewers analyzed digital recordings and/or transcriptions of focus group content to identify content themes. Five themes emerged from focus group participants: program design, developing nursing expertise, program impact on the unit, future expectations, and communication. Comments pertaining to each theme have been used to guide program improvements and offer new insights for residency programs in acute and critical care. (Adams et al., 2015).

Innovation to Improve Care

Goal: To utilize, develop, and translate nursing research to improve patient care

Outcome/exemplar: Reducing hospital-acquired pressure ulcers

The challenge: Hospital-acquired pressure ulcers (HAPU) have been recognized as complications that are generally preventable and associated with increased morbidity, mortality, and cost of care. In 2006, the total estimated cost of care for Stage 3 and Stage 4 pressure ulcers in the United States was $11 billion/year (Federal Register, 2008). Therefore, in 2007, the Centers for Medicare and Medicaid Services (CMS) identified Stage 3 and 4 pressure ulcers as "never events," or medical errors that should never occur. In 2008, CMS implemented nonpayment for treatment (Russo, Steiner, & Spector, 2008).

The response: The MGH Department of Nursing conducts quarterly pressure ulcer prevalence surveys with results reported to the National Database of Nursing Quality Indicators (NDNQI) and a statewide repository of quality metrics, Patient Care Link. Between September 2012 and June 2013, the quarterly pressure ulcer (PU) prevalence surveys demonstrated that one (4.3%) to five (23%) patients with PUs per quarter had undergone cardiac surgery (CS). The length of the surgery ranged from 3 to cumulative 16 hours during multiple surgical procedures.

A novel approach to prevent PUs from prolonged immobilization was spearheaded by our organizational clinical nurse specialist (CNS) in wound prevention, who is also a nurse scientist. CNS investigated the use of a pressure redistribution surface pad that uses a patented microprocessor and dynamic waveform analysis software to adjust internal air density based on mass and surface area. The end result is a support medium with less molecular density than the supported body, maintaining normal tissue symmetry (Biologics Pressure Relief Systems, 2014).

Evaluation: Between 1 September 2013 and 30 November 2013, a research study was conducted to determine whether the pad reduces PU incidence following CS. During this period, 398 patients underwent CS (coronary artery bypass graft aortic valve replacement, mitral valve replacement, thoracic aortic procedures, CABG plus VR lung transplant heart transplant) using the pad. The duration of the procedures was shortest for CABG and longest for thoracic aortic repair. During the study using the pads, the incidence of new pressure ulcers was 0%, indicating that they contribute to prevention of tissue deformation and consequent deep tissue injury in a subset of patients who are at very high risk of PU. Implications for practice include the expanded use of the pads for other patients at high risk for pressure ulcer development.

Scholarship and Dissemination

Goal: To share evidence to improve practice locally, nationally, and internationally

Outcome/exemplar: International symposia

The challenge: Our commitment extends beyond our own institution, with a responsibility to share our evidence to improve practice locally, nationally, and internationally. Members of the Institute for Patient Care consistently publish their outcomes in peer-reviewed journals and publications; are invited speakers for local, national, and international conferences; and serve as expert consultants on clinical practice, research, and EBP and education.

The response: Since the evolution of the institute, two international symposiums have been held, with a third under development in 2015 to spread the knowledge generated in our practice environment and share the lessons learned. The first, in 2011, Strategies for Creating and Sustaining a Professional Practice Environment, focused on strategies to develop and sustain professional practice. Past presentations have included the transformational power of nursing leadership, strategic planning and evaluation as essentials to sustainable change, specific scalable and translatable best practices such as an evidence-based approach to fall prevention, patient-family and provider partnerships, and an interdisciplinary model for shared decision-making. The second symposium, in 2013, Innovation in Care Delivery: Advancing a Professional Practice Environment, explored the changes we have experienced from conception, design, implementation, and evaluation of our innovation units, a new care delivery model with the potential to improve care, reduce costs, and increase patient and family satisfaction. A highlight of the symposium was the session devoted to a new role, the attending registered nurse (Ives Erickson, Ditomassi, & Adams, 2012). Pioneers in this role spoke eloquently about their increased ability to prevent gaps in care by establishing closer collaborative relationships with patients and families, serving as the care coordinator among multiple disciplines to foster continuity of care and utilizing evidence-based strategies such as discharge phone calls to improve patient outcomes.

Evaluation: Not only was the Innovation in Care Delivery Symposium a great success, it also validated our conviction that there *is* a way to make healthcare better.

There *is* a way to make care more efficient, affordable, and accessible. We've unlocked the door to a new realm of innovative thinking, and others are as eager to exploit the possibilities as we are.

Awards and Recognition

Goal: To create a framework for professional recognition and advancement

Outcome/exemplar: Clinical recognition program

The challenge: The clinical recognition program provides a way to formally recognize professional staff for their clinical expertise. Through the program, clinical staff from six disciplines in PCS analyze their own practice and can seek recognition for the level of practice that they have achieved. These disciplines include nursing, occupational therapy, physical therapy, respiratory therapy, social work, and speech-language and swallowing disorders. Two additional disciplines are currently preparing to join the program: chaplaincy and child life specialists.

The response: The clinical recognition program reflects the work of many clinicians in PCS who researched the field of skill acquisition and, in particular, studied the work of Dreyfus & Dreyfus (1986) and Benner (1984). They met with groups of MGH clinicians and examined narratives (stories of clinical practice) written by MGH staff. Through the committee's work, a picture of MGH practice emerged and is described through themes and levels of practice.

Evaluation: Four themes and four levels of practice were identified. The initial three levels used to analyze a clinician's practice are the clinician-patient relationship, clinical knowledge and decision-making, and teamwork and collaboration. A fourth theme, movement, was identified for occupational therapy and physical therapy only. As they gain knowledge and integrate their clinical experiences, the way in which they practice within and across each theme evolves and matures.

The clinical recognition program describes criteria within each theme that define four levels of clinical practice: entry-level clinician, clinician, advanced clinician, and clinical scholar.

Participation in the last two levels of the program is voluntary. Advanced clinician and clinical scholars assemble a professional portfolio that includes a clinical narrative that describes their practice and illustrates how it meets the criteria for the level of recognition being sought. This portfolio is submitted to an interdisciplinary review board composed of advanced clinicians, clinical scholars, clinical specialists, and unit/departmental leaders for consideration. Clinicians seeking recognition at these levels also participate in an interview with members of the review board as part of the application process. As of January 2015, there are 369 advanced clinicians and 162 clinical scholars who exemplify professional practice.

Workforce Diversity

Goal: To support minority nursing students and facilitate successful transition to clinical practice

Outcome/exemplar: The Clinical Leadership Collaborative for Diversity in Nursing (CLCDN)

The challenge: The nursing profession has not kept pace with the changing demographics of this country (American Association of Colleges of Nursing [AACN], 2014).

The response: The CLCDN was developed through an academic-practice part-nership focused on supporting minority nursing students and facilitating their successful transition to clinical practice. A key program element is professional mentoring. Minority students and experienced nurse clinicians were paired in a mentorship dyad to help guide the student throughout the junior and senior year of school as well as the first year of employment.

Evaluation: The mentoring component of the project was evaluated through sur-veys in which mentors and mentees rated one another and offered open-ended comments on the program's impact. Mentees were rated highest by mentors on components that included professional manner, ability to communicate and get along with others, preparation for meetings, and fully utilizing their time with mentors. Aspects of mentors rated highest by mentees included warmth, encouragement, and willingness to listen; enthusiasm for nursing and how they sparked the mentee's interest; and clarity regarding expectations for mentees and how they pushed mentees to achieve high standards. In the open-ended comments, mentees consistently identified mentoring as the program's strongest component. Sixty-four minority students have participated with a zero rate of attrition and very low job turnover among graduates (Banister, Bowen-Brady, & Winfrey, 2014). As the demographics of the country continue to change, more diverse nurses will be needed to provide culturally competent care and address health disparities in minority populations.

Collaborative Decision-Making

Goal: To place authority, responsibility, and accountability for patient care with practicing clinicians

Outcome/exemplar: Collaborative Governance (CG)

The challenge: The need to involve all staff across PCS in collaborative governance (i.e., a decision-making process that places authority, responsibility, and accountability for patient care with practicing clinicians)

The response: CG is based on the belief that a shared vision and common goals lead to a highly committed and productive workforce, that participation is empowering, and that people will make appropriate decisions when sufficient knowledge is known and communicated (Patient Care Services Operating Plan, 2002). CG integrates approximately 400 clinical staff from nursing, physical therapy, occupational therapy, speech-language and swallowing disorders, social work, and other disciplines from across the hospital into the formal decision-making structure of PCS. With the support of leadership, these front-line clinicians stimulate, facilitate, generate, and disseminate knowledge that will improve patient care, enhance the environment, and shape their practice.

Evaluation: Since launching CG in 1997, much has changed in healthcare, technology, and the evolving needs of patients and families. In 2010, a redesign effort was initiated to better align the work of CG with the strategic goals of PCS and the hospital, regulatory readiness, and Magnet redesignation efforts. An informatics committee was added to reflect the explosion of technological advances, including, for example, the electronic medical record, wireless technologies, and smart pumps. With the increasing focus on quality metrics, specific committees were charged with reducing or eliminating specific nursing-sensitive indicators such as falls, pressure ulcer prevention, and restraint use. For several years, the CG champions have been surveyed, examining structural empowerment (Kanter, 1993) and power as knowing participation in change (Barrett, 1998). In the most recent survey of 228 participants, there was a continuation in positive scoring on work effectiveness, psychological empowerment, and participation in change. Qualitative data from the study captured the rich experiences of CG participation, including meaningful personal and professional growth; feelings of being known, valued, and trusted; and making positive contributions to practice.

International Influence

Goal: To improve global healthcare and to promote professional dialogue across cultures

Outcome/exemplar: Global nursing education

The challenge: International collaboration. Massachusetts General Hospital has a long tradition of serving people throughout the world. Founding physicians James Jackson and John Collins Warren wrote a circular letter on August 20, 1810, urging the establishment of a general hospital in Boston in which they asserted that "when in distress, every man becomes our neighbor" (MGH celebrates 200-year anniversary of the circular letter, 2010).

The response: The Massachusetts legislature, led by former U.S. President John Adams, agreed and granted a charter for the MGH stating that the hospital should serve citizens of other countries and provide comfort to "the whole family of man" (MGH celebrates 200-year anniversary of the Circular Letter, 2010). With this important historical legacy in mind, the Global Nursing Education Program was developed in 1995. This program provides an opportunity for nurses throughout the world to visit MGH and consult with expert nursing leaders and clinicians. The primary goals of the program are to improve global healthcare and to promote professional dialogue across cultures. An individualized learning curriculum is designed for each visitor to meet his or her learning objectives. Options for learning include clinical observation, leadership consultation, and didactic lectures.

Evaluation: The scope of the program varies widely from specialty-focused goals, such as critical-care nursing, wound care, and nursing in the Cancer Center, to more organizationally focused objectives, including a focus on the PPM, quality improvement and patient safety, and hospital management and leadership development. Since its inception, the program has hosted over 1,000 visitors from across the United States and around the world.

Ethics and End-of-Life Care

Goal: To respond and mitigate conflict in clinical situations of ethical conflict at end of life

Outcome/exemplar: Optimum Care Committee and Clinical Ethics Residency in Nursing (CERN)

The challenge: Advancing the work of Nursing Ethics at MGH

The response: Our nurse ethicist, who is one of the organization's clinical nurse specialists and a nurse scientist, serves as co-chair of the hospital's Optimum Care (Ethics) Committee. In this role, the nurse ethecist co-leads an interdisciplinary/professional ethics consultation committee (Courtwright et al., 2013), which primarily serves to respond and mitigate conflict in clinical situations at the end of life. Ethical consults can be requested by any clinician, patient, or family member. End-of-life conflict themes over the past several years have shifted from physicians being hesitant to "withhold and withdraw" life-sustaining treatment despite the wishes of patients and families (Cantor, 2001) to a general theme of surrogate/families continuing to request life-sustaining treatments when physicians, nurses, and allied health professionals notice that such life-sustaining treatments are burdening the patient without providing benefit (Ferrell, 2006, pp. 922–930).

In addition, the nurse ethicist developed, implemented, and evaluated a transformative learning program called the Clinical Ethics Residency for Nurses (Robinson et al., 2014). Based on her extensive experience with nurses and nurse leaders who face challenges in caring for patients and their families when ethical dilemmas arise and her desire to provide effective advocacy, she and her colleagues focused on developing moral agency, "the enhanced ability to act and bring about change" (Robinson et al., 2014). To increase their knowledge, competencies, and skills with this focus, educational content included values exploration, reflective time, communication techniques, role playing, simulation, and mentorship.

Evaluation: The nurse ethicist served as co-investigator with a physician-researcher to conduct a research project to fully describe the MGH experience in ethics consultations. A secure platform to track individual cases provides a robust database of consultations from which data can be exported to SPSS for analysis has been developed, tested, and adopted by the researchers. The overall goal in the research is to identify trends in consultation that can inform policy development and revision in our institution, as well as to lead to insights and development of interventions to work more effectively with surrogate decision-makers in cases where ethical conflict exists. In regards to CERN, 67 nurses participated in the program. Pre-post measures of moral distress, ethics knowledge, and self-efficacy showed statistically significant improvements.

Summary

The IPC is committed to generating and advancing knowledge development; supporting the development, integration, and translation of EBP; and preparing future leaders at the unit level and throughout the organization. As the work of the institute continues to expand and evolve, the future has limitless possibilities. It is anticipated that centers of clinical excellence involving staff development, research, and EBP will emerge and become focal areas for funding, research, professional advancement, and recognition. The visibility and influence of the IPC, its centers, and its programmatic initiatives are growing and gaining international recognition. Recently, the MGH embarked upon a 5-year strategic planning process. Representatives from the institute co-led and/or participated in many of the committees that focused on the future of education, research, clinical practice, and community health. Members of the IPC hold positions of influence on the three executive committees sanctioned by the MGH board of directors: the Executive Committee on Research, the Executive Committee on Education, and the Executive Committee on Community Health.

The IPC continues to expand its efforts to work together and forge innovation in healthcare delivery. The institute, through its centers and programs, collaborates with all disciplines to redefine processes, roles, and responsibilities to better serve patients' and our communities' overall healthcare needs in the most cost-effective manner. The IPC evaluates, informs, and celebrates quality care. It is an evolving framework for continuing our efforts to address the complexity of healthcare delivery. We are proud of how far we've come, but we have much more to do.

The author wishes to acknowledge the contributions of Jeffrey M. Adams, RN, PhD, Virginia Capasso, PhD, RN, R. Gino Chisari DNP, RN, Brian French, MS, RN-BC, Dorothy A. Jones, EdD, RN, FAAN, FNI, Jane Keefe MBA, RN, Ellen Robinson PhD, RN, and Mary Ellin Smith MSN, RN.

References

Adams, J. M., Alexander, G., Chisari, R. G., Banister, G., McAuley, M., Whitney, K., & Ives Erickson, J. (2015). Strengthening new graduate nurse residency programs in critical care: Recommendations from nurse residents and organizational stakeholders. *Journal of Continuing Education in Nursing, 46*(1), 41-48.

American Association of Colleges of Nursing (AACN). (2014). Fact sheet: Enhancing diversity in the nursing workforce. Retrieved from http://www.aacn.nche.edu/media-relations/diversityFS.pdf

Banister, G., Bowen-Brady, H., & Winfrey, M. E. (2014). Using career nurse mentors to support minority nursing students and facilitate their transition to practice. *Journal of Professional Nursing, 30*(4), 317-325.

Barrett, E. M. (1998). A nursing theory of power for nursing practice. In J. Riehl (Ed.), *Conceptual models for nursing practice* (3rd ed). Norwalk, CT: Appleton & Lange.

Benner, P. (1984). *From novice to expert: Excellence and power in clinical nursing practice.* Menlo Park, CA: Addison-Wesley Publishing Company.

Biologics Pressure Relief Systems (2014). Retrieved from http://www.biologics900t.com/news.html

Cantor, N. L. (2001). Twenty-five years after Quinlan: A review of the jurisprudence of death and dying. *Journal of Law, Medicine & Ethics, 29,* 182-196.

Courtwright, A. M., Brackett, S., Cist, A., Cremens, M. C., Krakauer, E. L, & Robinson, E. M. (2013). The changing composition of a hospital ethics committee: A tertiary care center's experience. *HEC Forum* DOI 0.1007/s10730-013-9218-0.

Dreyfus, H.L., & Dreyfus, S. E. (1986). *Mind over machine the power of human intuition and expertise in the era of the computer.* New York: The Free Press.

Federal Register 73(161). August 19, 2008 Rules and Regulations. Retrieved from http:// edocket.access.gpo.gov/2008/pdf/E8-17914.pdf

Ferrell, B. R. (2006). Understanding the moral distress of nurses witnessing medically futile care. *Oncology Nursing Forum, 33*(5), 922-930.

Institute of Medicine (IOM). (2001). *Crossing the quality chasm: A new health system for the 21st century.* Washington, DC: The National Academies Press.

Institute of Medicine. (2003) *Unequal Treatment: Confronting racial and ethnic disparities in health care.* Washington, DC: The National Academies Press.

Institute of Medicine (IOM). (2011). *The future of nursing: Leading change, advancing health.* Washington, DC: The National Academies Press.

Institute of Medicine. (2014). *Integrating research and practice: Health system leaders working toward high-value care: workshop summary.* Washington, DC: The National Academies Press.

Ives Erickson, J. (2006). 2006 Patient care services annual report, *MGH Patient Care Services.*

Ives Erickson, J., & Ditomassi, M. (2012). Professional Practice Model: strategies for translating models into practice. In Ives Erickson, J., Jones, D., & Ditomassi, M. (Eds.), *Fostering Nurse-Led Care Professional Practice for the Bedside from Massachusetts General Hospital.* Indianapolis, IN: Sigma Theta Tau International.

Ives Erickson, J., Ditomassi, M., & Adams, J. M. (2012). Attending registered nurse: An innovative role to manage between the spaces. *Nursing Economics, 30*(5), 282-287.

Ives Erickson, J., Ditomassi, M., & Jones, D. (2008). Interdisciplinary institute for patient care: Advancing clinical excellence. *Journal of Nursing Administration, 38*(6), 308-314.

Ives Erickson, J., Ditomassi, M & Jones, D. (2013). *Fostering Nurse-Led Care at the Bedside: Professional Practice for the Bedside Leader from Massachusetts General Hospital.* Indianapolis, IN: Sigma Theta Tau International.

Kanter, R. M. (1993). *Men and women in the corporation* (2nd ed.). New York: Basic Books

Massachusetts General Hospital. (2009). Mission, Credo and Boundaries. Retrieved from http://library.partners.org/MGH1/webserver/custom/trovedemoframeset.asp

MGH celebrates 200-year anniversary of the circular letter. (2010, August 20). *Hotline.*

Patient Care Services operating plan. 2002. MGH Patient Care Services.

Robinson, E. M., Lee, S. M., Zollfrank, A., Jurchak, M., Frost, D., & Grace, P. (2014). Enhancing moral agency: Clinical ethics residency for nurses. *Hastings Center Report, 44*(5), 12-20.

Russo, C. A., Steiner, C., & Spector, W. (2008). Hospitalizations related to pressure ulcers, 2006. HCUP Statistical Brief #64. Retrieved from http://www.hcup-us.ahrq.gov/reports/statbriefs/sb64

Senge, P.M. 1990. *The Fifth Discipline.* London: Century Business.

Chapter 3

Promoting Nursing Research Through the Yvonne L. Munn Center

–Dorothy A. Jones, EdD, RN, FAAN, FNI

The Yvonne L. Munn Center for Nursing Research (Munn Center) offers nurses an opportunity to participate in the development, testing, utilization, and evaluation of nursing research. By fostering and supporting an organizational climate that promotes scholarly inquiry, patient- and family-centered care is enhanced, and the professional practice environment (PPE) is optimized (Jones, 2009).

The Munn Center is a presence within Patient Care Services (PCS), the Institute for Patient Care (IPC), and the Massachusetts General Hospital (MGH) community of scholars. Doctorally prepared nurses and staff at MGH serve on interdisciplinary committees across the MGH research enterprise, actively engaging in the advancement of knowledge through research and inquiry. The continued development of the Munn Center has resulted in the expansion of nursing scholarship as well as the creation of new partnerships and collaborations across disciplines. These research initiatives have provided a forum to explore and uncover new knowledge and articulate nursing's impact on high-quality patient/family care outcomes.

The Munn Center was named after former Associate General Director and Director of Nursing Yvonne L. Munn, whose tenure at MGH spanned from 1984 to 1993. Throughout her long and distinguished career, Mrs. Munn promoted family-focused, evidence-driven, research-based practice. Her commitment to excellence in nursing was enhanced by her commitment to research and discovery. The Munn Center was established through the leadership and commitment of Jeanette Ives Erickson, senior vice president for patient care and chief nurse. With the support of the MGH organizational leadership, Ives Erickson was able to provide the resources needed to foster the growth of the Munn Center as an important strategy to inform patient care, shape and influence professional development, foster new opportunities to improve health, enhance recovery, accelerate healing, and advance patient/family-focused, relationship-based care (Ives Erickson, Ditomassi, & Jones, 2013).

This chapter focuses on the mission, goals, infrastructure, and innovative strategies in place within the Munn Center to advance nursing research and discovery. More importantly, the successes experienced throughout the implementation of the Munn Center and the development of an environment where nurse clinicians and scholars can create and validate evidence and advance a research agenda are explained and examples discussed.

Munn Center and the IPC

As discussed in Chapter 2, "Creating an Infrastructure that Enhances Professional Practice and Patient Care Services," the Munn Center is one of four centers within the IPC. The leadership of the Munn Center works collaboratively with all centers to achieve the goals of the IPC and enhance the synergistic relationship between and among all centers.

The Munn Center is housed within the IPC to foster the development, implementation, evaluation, and translation of knowledge gained through clinical inquiry to improve patient care. Through the generosity of Mrs. Yvonne L. Munn and the support of Peter Slavin, MD, MGH president, much has been accomplished to advance a nursing research agenda that promotes the growth of nursing science and offers new opportunities for collaboration. The creation of a culture of inquiry optimizes patient care and enhances nurses' satisfaction with the PPE (Duffy, 2013). The official dedication of the Munn Center, held on May 7, 2008, acknowledged MGH's commitment to nursing research and inter-disciplinary research collaboration.

The articulation of a research agenda to develop, test, refine, and extend knowledge directly influences the culture of patient care, increases the visibility of professional practice and uses evidence to shape care delivery. Currently, this work is occurring in several focal areas, including workforce evaluation, symptom management, and evidence-based practice. The use of multiple research methodologies are used measure the impact of clinical inquiry on care outcomes.

The Munn Center focuses on:

- Promoting nursing science through creating an infrastructure and support needed to advance a nursing research agenda

- Collaborating and leading investigations that foster staff knowledge and experience around the conduct of research and promote the integration of new knowledge to enhance the delivery of safe, quality, cost-effective patient care

From the acquisition of a physical space to the coordination of research efforts across the MGH community, the Munn Center has enabled nurses to partner with other nurses and colleagues in other disciplines to promote knowledge across the patient and family's health-illness experience.

Munn Center Goals

The Munn Center is focused on building knowledge to improve care and enhance the practice environment of care. Generating, testing, and refining knowledge through research helps to advance nursing science and produce evidence that informs care across settings and populations. The Munn Center is guided by a set of goals responsive to the MGH as an organization, PCS, and the IPC, as follows:

- Advance a nursing research agenda at MGH and beyond.

- Create a culture of inquiry that stimulates discovery.

- Develop an infrastructure, including committees and grant funding processes, to implement the goals of the Munn Center.

- Implement mentoring strategies to promote an active research agenda for all nurses in PCS to be active participants.

- Generate new partnerships and funding mechanisms within MGH and with external funding sources.

- Disseminate research in scholarly journals and present findings at scholarly meetings.

- Design strategies to promote the development, use, and translation of evidence into practice.

- Generate original research that extends and refines nursing existing nursing knowledge essential to improving patient care.

- Collaborate with other centers in the IPC to enhance the work of the institute.

- Actively participate in Executive Committee on Research (ECOR) and the MGH Research Council to develop new collaborative opportunities across disciplines.

- Continue to accelerate research in core areas of focus: care of the elderly, ethics, symptom management, workforce evaluation, and complementary healing interventions to promote healing and recovery.

- Work in partnership with other groups to advance the strategic mission of PCS.

- Actively contribute data and examples of evidence to achieve Magnet® redesignation.

The Research Center Team

Since its inception, the Munn Center has assembled a team of nurse scientists and staff prepared to assist MGH nursing staff, faculty, students, and others in the coordination, conduct, and dissemination of research initiatives to advance nursing knowledge and improve care delivery.

Building a research team has been guided by the goals and mission of PCS and the MGH organization. The development of a Munn Center team reflects the influence of nursing leadership, the goals of the IPC, and the members of the Munn Center team. The success of the center is not only manifested in its processes and products but also through its influence on a practice culture across PCS that values inquiry, discovery, and creativity. The members of the current Munn Center team and their roles are as follows:

- Director of the Munn Center (also a senior nurse scientist)

- Nurse scientists (both full- and part-time)

- Grant manager (part-time; assists with budget planning, manages grant tracker for Magnet Recognition Program® documentation)

- Postdoctoral fellows and research assistants (per diem staff; work with Munn Center staff on special projects)

- Statistics consultant (part-time)

- Administrative assistant (full-time)

- Grant developer/writer/Qualtrics administrator/data analysis (part-time)

- Partnership with director of the MGH Research Center; use of added statistical services and grant development resources available

- Additional personnel associated with grants, added for projects only

Staff holds both full-time and part-time appointments in the center. They occupy physical space in the center, with additional meeting space and room for research assistants and funded grant personnel.

Opportunities for Nurse Scientists

The development of the nurse scientist and senior nurse scientist roles has been a critical addition to accomplishing the Munn Center goals. Opportunities for involvement in activities within the center, committee leadership, mentoring staff and students, as well as engaging in the development and implementation and evaluation of funded and unfunded research investigations are facilitated by the Munn Center team members.

The job descriptions for both the nurse scientist and senior nurse scientist are:

- **Nurse scientist:** This nurse is a doctorally prepared nurse researcher early in a career in research. This individual has clinical expertise and specific area of nursing inquiry that can be further studied and developed. This individual is expected to continue to develop and advance a program of research, seek funding, contribute to nursing knowledge development; participate in mentoring activities, serve as a reviewer (grant or abstract), promote the use and integration of research into practice and beyond, consult with staff, collaborate with other researchers, and disseminate research nationally.

- **Senior nurse scientist:** This nurse is an accomplished nurse scholar, a leader in the discipline and funded researcher known for a body of inquiry or area of research focus. The senior nurse scientist mentors students and other researchers, has disseminated work internationally, publishes extensively in high-impact journals, and collaborates on research initiatives across disciplines and settings.

In addition, the work of over 50 doctorally prepared nurses within the PCS and the MGH community is linked to the Munn Center's infrastructure and offers an opportunity to engage other nurse scholars in clinical inquiry and discovery.

The Munn Center team's growth continues to be affected by the staff's visibility and responsiveness to PCS' and MGH's organizational research agendas. The Munn Center team has successfully built an infrastructure that advances nursing research within a practice setting and promotes nurses' participation in the conduct of research. As external funding opportunities continue to expand, additional staff can be hired to implement and evaluate a specific research investigation.

Research Opportunities for All Nurses

By engaging all nurses in the research enterprise, the Munn Center has its presence within the MGH research community. Over the years, the Munn Center has identified multiple opportunities for staff to be involved in research and inquiry. The ability to engage all staff in research and provide opportunities for them to participate in clinical inquiry has increased staff's research activity. This process has been cultivated over several years, and many staff have engaged the Munn Center staff in assisting them with implementing initiatives such as grant writing, writing for publication, abstract writing, and preparing presentations. Table 3.1 provides examples of how nurses with different research expertise may choose to engage in research activities.

TABLE 3.1   Research Opportunities Available to All Nursing Staff

ROLE	ACTIVITY
Clinical nurses	Use nursing knowledge to inform practice decisions and develop scholarship to disseminate knowledge and research experiences.
	Seek mentoring to identify researchable topics, clinical questions, and related research studies needed to conduct clinical inquiry.
	Participate actively in relevant collaborative governance committees and evidence-based practice initiatives.
	Obtain funding to support clinical investigations through Yvonne L. Munn Research Awards.
Master-degreed nurses	Stimulate staff participation in the development and conduct of evidence-based practice and research investigations.
	Seek mentoring by more senior researchers to advance one's own research and begin to publish.
	Participate in relevant collaborative governance and evidence-based practice initiatives as a leader.
	Seek research funding through the annual Yvonne L. Munn Research Awards and other internal funding opportunities.

continues

TABLE 3.1 *continued*

ROLE	ACTIVITY
Doctoral students	Participate in the Doctoral Forum to network research interest groups and begin publishing.
	Design flexible schedules to support academic advancement.
Doctorally prepared nurses	Develop, test, and evaluate the impact of new knowledge and research evidence to inform care delivery and workforce issues.
	Mentor Yvonne L. Munn Nursing Research awardees.
	Seek funding and support to advance a program of research through the Yvonne L. Munn Postdoctoral Fellowship and by accessing external funding sources.
	Strengthen opportunities within the Doctoral Forum to develop and pursue a program of research resulting in publications and funding.
	Generate research to inform care redesign and improve cost-effective, high-quality, safe, and efficient patient/family-centric care through research.
External faculty	Mentor doctorally prepared nurses and staff in clinical research activities to build a program of research.
	Disseminate research findings and expand research activities with staff and members of an interdisciplinary healthcare team.
	Contribute knowledge to the advancement of nursing research by conducting clinical investigations that promote nursing inquiry and knowledge development.

Opportunities for External Faculty Nurse Scientists

The appointment of faculty as external nurse scientists to the Munn Center has been an effective strategy to expand research opportunities for staff and faculty. The application and appointment process of external faculty nurse scientists to the Munn Center has helped to enhance clinical and academic partnerships, expanded mentoring opportunities, helped faculty access clinical research sites, accelerated Institutional Review Board (IRB) access, and contributed to advancing a research agenda. Appointments of external faculty nurse scientists to the Munn Center are not funded positions. Faculty who are appointed to the Munn Center may have access to space, computers, and other resources to support research activities while they are on the MGH campus.

Currently, more than 65 national and international external faculty nurse scientists have been appointed to the Munn Center. Their presence continues to expand the research mission and goals of the Munn Center and PCS. Qualifications for appointments include a master's degree in nursing and a doctorate in nursing or a related field, licensure as a registered nurse, and faculty appointment to an accredited university. Each application is reviewed on an individual basis, and appointments are made according to criteria established by the Munn Center. Faculty members interested in an appointment are invited to submit a letter of request along with their curriculum vitae to the Munn Center. The expectations of this appointment are as follows:

- Participate in the mentoring of doctorally prepared nurses and staff in clinical research activities in the process of building a program of research.

- Disseminate research findings and expand research activities with staff and members of an interdisciplinary healthcare team.

- Contribute to research goals of the organization by helping to advance the research agenda of future scholars at MGH.

- Meet with staff from the Munn Center in a variety of forums, including a "think tank" and the Munn Research Awards review committee.

- Participate in Doctoral Forum activities and, when appropriate, present research at Grand Rounds. (For more information about Grand Rounds, see Chapter 6, "Promoting Nursing Research in a Multidisciplinary Organization.")

- Contribute knowledge to the advancement of nursing research at MGH by engaging in and promoting nursing inquiry and knowledge development.

An added outcome of the external faculty appointments had been the development of new partnerships with academic settings and medical centers internationally. Several scholars from within the United States, China, Japan, Spain, and Brazil have had appointments in the Munn Center as postdoctoral fellows, working with the Munn Center staff and participating in research and scholarly publications with other nurse scientists. Their time in the Munn Center is supported by sponsoring universities and clinical settings. Their appointments range from 1 month to 1 year in duration.

Munn Center Activities

Staff members of the Munn Center engage in multiple activities. Many occur on a regular basis (e.g., team and Munn Center committee meetings), whereas others occur in response to an organizational request (e.g., evaluation of the Professional Practice Model [PPM]). All activities are led or co-led by a member of the Munn Center team so that there is consistent feedback to the Munn Center leadership around implementation and sustainability of committee and center goals.

Team Meetings

The Munn Center holds regular team meetings on a monthly basis throughout the year. These meetings are chaired by the director of the Munn Center. The administrative assistant takes minutes and prepares them for review by meeting participants. The executive director of the IPC is invited to attend team meetings and receives all agendas and previous minutes. Team documents are stored and become a part of future Magnet evidence.

In addition to the regular team meetings, the quarterly team meetings are expanded to include not only the Munn team but also Munn committee leaders and groups across PCS and linked to facilitating Munn Center activities. All team meetings occur on the first Thursday of the month and last approximately 2 hours. A sample agenda from a quarterly meeting is provided in the following sidebar.

EXAMPLE OF A QUARTERLY MUNN RESEARCH TEAM MEETING AGENDA

1.0   *Minutes from last quarterly Munn Research Team meeting.*

2.0   *Announcements.*

3.0   *Institute Ops: Update monthly meeting with directors for centers within IPC.*

4.0   *Munn Center: Updates and announcements to include personnel changes/ news, and visitor updates, important meetings, studies in progress, grant opportunities, and publications.*

5.0   *Magnet Recognition Program®: Updates and planning to include data collection and storage of evidence; grant tracker updates.*

6.0   *Policy development and implementation—includes information on website and dissemination site plan.*

7.0   *Innovation: Updates focus on implementation and evaluation research strategies.*

8.0   *IRB updates: Include a report from committee membership within and external to Munn Center.*

9.0   *ECOR updates: Examples include meeting with medical director, participation in Research Council, PCORI grant follow-up, updates from Harvard Catalyst reviewers.*

10.   *Communication with nurse researchers, Munn Center presentation at next council meeting, Clinical Research Day Poster Award.*

11.   *Nursing Research Grand Rounds—includes updates, multidisciplinary involvement; communication of presentations in Caring Headlines and video on website.*

12.   *Connell Nursing Research Scholars—includes program updates, development updates, new opportunities.*

13.   *Budget: Updates to include grant submissions, policies, grant tracker review, and current funding.*

14.   *Grant submission process—includes new policies reviewed re: grant submission process and web update.*

15. *Munn Pre-/Postdoctoral Fellowship: Updates by committee leaders.*

16. *Doctoral Forum: Updates by committee leaders, monthly and annual agenda review, websites and outreach to internal doctoral faculty and external faculty nurse scientists.*

17. *Munn Awards and Review: Updates by committee leaders to include educational planning; pre- and post-award, mentoring policies, website updates, and publications and presentations reviewed.*

18. *Research Expo—Annual Research Day: Updates by committee leaders includes abstract preparation and review, poster development, communication plan, and research program.*

19. *Other updates: from Librarian, Clinical Research Center; clinical nurse researchers; CNSRTF—Clinical special project; and other special projects.*

20. *Other topics.*

21. *Next meeting.*

Budget Administration

The Munn Center has its own budget. It is managed by the director in concert with the executive director of the IPC. The Munn Center also has a grant manager (GM), whose responsibilities include the following:

- Maintains oversight of center expenses and meets with the leadership to review budget funds and expenses

- Maintains a grant tracker that lists of all grant activities and monitors all accounts over the course of funding

- Meets with each principal investigator (PI) to review budgets and address issues around the completion of required grant reporting

- Monitors all grant activity and grant compliance for funded research initiatives

- Provides a budget update at monthly meetings and holds additional meetings with the Munn Center director to review the budget and expenditures

- Meets with any staff involved with a grant submission to prepare and revise budgets

- Submits all grants directly from the Munn Center to the Office of Grants and Contracts and then by Grants and Contracts to the respective funding agency

Munn Center Communication and Committee Structure

The Munn Center is able to accomplish many of its goals through a network of communication activities with PCS, IPC, and a committee infrastructure. Information from the Munn Center projects and initiatives are published on a regular basis in MGH publications (e.g., *Caring Headlines* and *Hotline*), the Munn Center brochure, and email. In addition, the Munn Center website at www.mghpcs.org/MunnCenter contains an invaluable amount of information and is updated by Munn Center staff on a regular basis.

A large component of Munn Center work is conducted through an active committee infrastructure. Each committee is led and or co-led by staff within PCS. Generally, these leaders are doctorally prepared (and at times masters prepared) nurse clinicians who work in collaboration with the Munn Center to advance specific components of Munn Center research agenda. The committees meet on a regular basis with Munn Center staff to discuss updates and review progress toward achieving goals. Committee leaders also provide a report at the quarterly Munn team meetings. Co-leading a committee offers staff an opportunity to participate and guide nursing research and helps to advance a culture of inquiry among nurses. A brief discussion of each committee and their activities is provided in the follow sections.

Munn Awards Committees

Several internal annual research awards are given to nursing staff annually on a competitive basis. Each award is led by a committee that works throughout the year to provide the required mentoring, grant application development, grant submission and review process, grant implementation, and reporting and dissemination of research findings. Generally, two co-leaders of the awards committees selected from across PCS accomplish this work. The Munn Center works with the committee leaders to assist with this work as needed. The Munn Nursing Research Awards, the Munn Pre/Postdoctoral Award, and the Connell Nursing Research Awards are examples of award committees. Information about each award can be accessed on the Munn Center website (www.mghpcs.org/ MunnCenter).

The Munn Nursing Research Awards

The Munn Nursing Research Awards are given annually to MGH clinical nurses (non-doctorally prepared) for the purpose of engaging the clinical nurse in a mentored research experience. The intent of each proposal is to support and advance PCS's annual strategic goals and promote the implementation of the PCS PPM. The Munn Nursing Research Awards program focuses on three main categories of activity:

- **Original research:** The purpose of research is to generate new knowledge within the broader scientific community to produce knowledge that is generalizable beyond the study sample.

- **Evidence-based practice (EBP):** The purpose of EBP is to evaluate evidence along a continuum to identify the strongest or best evidence to guide nursing practice within an organizational setting and with a specific patient population.

- **Performance improvement (PI) project:** The purpose of a PI project is to improve internal processes and practices within a specific patient group or organization.

Applicants seeking an Yvonne L. Munn Nursing Research Award must be a registered nurse, in a clinical nurse role, and working at least 20 hours per week as a permanent employee at MGH. Part-time nurses are encouraged to work collaboratively with a full-time co-PI. A doctorally prepared MGH nurse serves as a mentor to each research team to provide guidance and oversight and to enhance the rigor of the investigation. All application proposals for a Munn Nursing Research Award are prepared and revised with center support.

A formal review of all Munn Awards submitted is completed online by a selection committee that includes representation from within the MGH community as well as appointed external faculty nurse scientists from schools of nursing across the Massachusetts. Evaluation criteria for the Munn Research Awards include the following:

Title of proposal

Abstract (500 words, maximum)

Introduction (1 page, maximum)

Background (identify gap in knowledge) and significance (2 pages, maximum)

Purpose/statement (2 sentences, maximum)

Aims with research question (1 page, maximum)

Methodology (3 pages, maximum)

Data analysis (1 page, maximum)

Potential contributions (1 page, maximum)

Budget and attachments (no page limit)

All submissions are reviewed with proposal authors, and the winners are announced on Nursing Research Day during Nurse Recognition Week. Small grant funding is awarded to meet budgeted goals. Completed studies are presented to an interdisciplinary audience throughout the year at quarterly Munn Nursing Research Grand Rounds. Following the announcement of the Munn awardees, both funded and unfunded staff meet with Munn Center staff to review plans for project implementation or resubmission. Paula Restrepo, an awardee in 2012, said, "The Munn Award provided me the resources and opportunity that empowered me to improve patient care for our patients." (Munn Center Nursing Research Award, n.d.). Examples of past recipients and their projects are found in Table 3.2.

TABLE 3.2 Examples of Staff Research and the Munn Research

YEAR	PROJECT	RESEARCH TEAM
2004–5	Music as a Therapeutic Intervention in Care of Neuromedical & Neurosurgical Patients	Alyona Runyans, MA, RN; Whitney Foster, BA, RN; Anastatia Michaelidis, RN; Jennifer O'Neill, BSN, RN; Marion Phipps, MS, RN Diane L. Carroll, PhD, RN, FAAN, (mentor)
2004–5	Psychological Insulin Resistance: A Study of Patients' Attitudes, Perceptions, and Fears	Mary E. Larkin, BSN, RN, CDE Virginia Capasso, PhD, APRN, BC (mentor)
2007	Evaluation of Basic Arrhythmia Knowledge Retention and Clinical Application by Registered Nurses	Laura Sumner, Med, RN, MBA, MSN, APRN-BC, ONC; Sheila Burke, BSN, RN, CCRN; Mary McAdams, BSN, RN-C; Lin-Ti Chang, MSN, RN-C, APRN-BC, CCRN Dorothy A. Jones, EdD, RN, FAAN, FNI (mentor)
2008	Exploring Women's Lived Experiences of Endocrine-Based Oral Chemotherapy for Breast Cancer	Loren Winters, MSN, RNC Dorothy A. Jones, EdD, RN, FAAN, FNI (mentor)
2008	Effects of Sensory Interventions on an Inpatient Psychiatric Unit: A Pilot Study	Christina Gulliver, MS, RN, APRN, CS Patricia Martin Arcari, PhD, RN (mentor)
2010	Family Members' Perceptions of Most Helpful Interventions During End-of-Life Care of a Loved One	Principal investigator: Julie Cronin, BSN, OCN Paul Arnstein, PhD, RN (mentor)

YEAR	PROJECT	RESEARCH TEAM
2010	The Impact of Death and Dying in the Intensive Care Unit on New Graduate Nurses	Principal investigators: Tara Tehan, MSN, MBA, RN; Mary Guanci, RN, MSN, CNRN Donna Perry, PhD, RN (mentor)
2011	Patients' Experiences of Hatha Yoga During Autologous Hematopoietic Stem Cell Transplant	Principal investigator: Jennifer Brock, BSN, RN Anne-Marie Barron, PhD, RN, CS (mentor)
2012	Comparison of Temporal Artery to Pulmonary Artery Thermistor Temperatures in Hyperthermic Patients	Principal investigator: Cynthia Finn, BS, RN Co-investigators: Donna Furlong, RN; Diane Gay, RN; Christine Gryglik, RN; Vivian Donahue, MSN, RN Diane L. Carroll, PhD, RN, FAAN (mentor)
2013	Understanding Determinates of Physical Restraint Use Among Critical-Care Patients: An Exploratory Study of Nurses	Principal investigator: Jeanne Dolan, MSN, RN Sara Dolan Looby, PhD, ANP-BC, FAAN (mentor)
2013	The Effects of Connective Tissue Massage on Pain in Post-Cesarean Section Primiparous Women	Louise T. Doyle, BSN, RNC-OB, HNB-BC Colleen Simonelli, RN, PhD (mentor)
2013	Nursing Assessment of Predictors of Diabetic Ketoacidosis Readmission in Adult Patients	Kerry B. Grennan, RN, ANP-BC, CDE Stephanie Ball, DSN, RN, CCRN, CCNS (mentor)

The Munn Pre/Postdoctoral Fellowship in Nursing Research

The development of the Yvonne L. Munn Doctoral Fellowship in Nursing Research (pre- and postdoctoral) is designed to create research opportunities in two ways:

- To expand doctorally prepared nurses' ability to complete publications and initiate grant funding activities

- To support doctoral candidates who are actively working to complete the dissertation

The overarching goal of the fellowship is to provide time and resources needed to accelerate research inquiry.

Each fellowship subsidizes up to 400 hours of the fellow's practice time and provides limited funding for related expenses over a 2-year period. Selection criteria for the award are developed by the Yvonne L. Munn Doctoral Fellowship in Nursing Research Committee and the Munn Center. Proposals must meet IRB criteria for proposals. A call for applications occurs annually.

The predoctoral fellowship is designed for a doctoral student who is currently a PhD candidate in dissertation phase of his or her program. It is anticipated that the fellowship will accelerate completion of the dissertation. The Munn postdoctoral fellowship is designed to facilitate the completion of an article or articles from the applicant's dissertation or promote the development of a pilot study.

Applications for these awards are available on the Munn Center website (www.mghpcs.org/MunnCenter) and completed applications are sent to the Fellowship Committee co-leaders. A Fellowship Review Committee participates in the selection process. The award is announced at Nursing Research Day. Follow-up implementation plans are reviewed and monitored by Munn Center staff. Publications and presentations at Nursing Research Grand Rounds are expected of each fellow.

Connell Nursing Research Scholars Award

The Connell Nursing Research Scholars (CNRS) program is the result of generous funding from the William F. Connell family to advance nursing research. The award is designed to advance postdoctoral nursing research by supporting a cohort of nurse scholars to advance a program of research. The award provides each scholar with protected clinical time (2 days or 16 hours), mentoring by Munn staff, as well as a national scholar in the field and support for traveling and dissemination of research. Participation in the CNRS program provides each scholar the time and active mentoring needed to generate and extend knowledge and advance interdisciplinary research collaboration. CNRS applications are designed to reflect each scholar's research accomplishments and expertise within the strategic priorities of PCS and the MGH organizational mission.

An advisory team consisting of MGH staff from across disciplines and external nurse scholars review applications and select CNRSs. A detailed application process developed by the Munn Center staff is posted on the Munn Center website. New Connell Scholars are announced to the MGH community during Nurse Recognition Week. Information about each scholar is disseminated in publications such as *Caring Headlines* as well as other communication venues. Since the inception of the program, nine scholars from the available cohort of doctorally prepared nurse researchers within PCS have been selected to participate in the funded postdoctoral CNRS program. All Connell Scholars meet regularly with Munn Staff to discuss their progress as well as research design, grant writing, and so on. As of this writing, outcomes of the CNRS program include additional grant submissions, numerous publications, international presentations, and national networking opportunities within the nursing and multidisciplinary research community. You can find a complete discussion of this program in Chapter 7, "Researching, Mentoring, and Developing Postdoctoral Scholars."

Clinical Nurse Specialist Research Task Force

The Clinical Nurse Specialist Research Task Force (CNS RTF) is a subgroup of the larger cohort of MGH clinical nurse specialists who self-select to actively engage in research. Participants in this group work closely with the Munn Center leadership to advance a nursing research agenda that centers on the CNS's scope of work and initiatives that complement the strategic goals of PCS. The CNS RTF meets on a regular basis and addresses issues related to EBP, quality care, education, and professional development. The group has implemented research results to guide improvements in patient outcomes and tested innovative strategies to improve care and promote knowledge development.

For several years, this group has worked with the Munn Center on a project focusing on the commonly occurring nursing diagnoses across practice settings. This ongoing research has been funded by NANDA-I and results disseminated internationally. The findings from this work have informed the nursing diagnoses used in the patient electronic patient record and guided staff development and implementation of evidence-based initiatives, including the Wound Education Program, the Basic Respiratory Program, an Intermediate Respiratory Program, the Abuse Management Program, the MGH Tracheostomy Quality Team, and a diabetes education rollout. The work of the CNS RTF has been used to increase the knowledge of staff, patients, and families. Exposure to the CNS RTF has served to motivate CNS staff to actively participate in work around the electronic medical record and nursing documentation and increase their efforts around developing evidence-based projects.

The Doctoral Forum

The Doctoral Forum was developed to support the growth and development of nurse scientists through dialogue and discussion. The goal of this group is to stimulate inquiry; provide supportive critique to improve a publication, grant, or presentation; and offer feedback on grant proposals. In addition, the Doctoral Forum is a supportive, professional community of nurse scholars who collaborate to help advance individual programs of research and stimulate the development of interdisciplinary research teams to engage in the research process. Through networking with other doctorally prepared nurses at MGH, external faculty nurse scientists, and other research scholars, ideas can be explored, new knowledge shared, and creative inquiry stimulated. Nurses with their earned doctorates, faculty nurse scientists appointed to the Munn Center, and nurses enrolled in a doctoral program are members of this community of scholars.

The Doctoral Forum is co-led by a doctorally prepared member of the Munn Center staff. The meetings focus on discussions around specific research topics (e.g., research methods), publishing, and presentations. Other activities include manuscript review, participating in abstract reviews submitted for Nursing Research Day presentations, poster evaluation, judging for Nursing Research Day awards, and serving as mentor for Munn Award applicants. Future work will promote group collaboration, team building, and grant writing. Opportunities for creating networking opportunities outside of nursing and exploring the work of PhD and DNP members will be part of future agenda items.

Harvard Catalyst

Harvard Catalyst brings together the knowledge, research, and clinical expertise of Harvard University and its affiliates and partners to reduce the burden of human illness. Members of the Harvard Catalyst include Harvard University and its 10 schools and 18 academic healthcare centers. Additional members include the Boston College School of Nursing, MIT, Harvard Pilgrim Health Care, and numerous community partners. The Harvard Clinical and Translational Science Center is dedicated to improving human health by enabling collaboration among these groups around the research enterprise. The Harvard Catalyst is a member of the NIH-funded Clinical and Translational Science Award Consortium and is dedicated to building a multidisciplinary research agenda through collaborative research activities, sharing resources, and developing funding through active grant development.

Nurses from the Munn Center, as well as from MGH PCS, are members of the Harvard Catalyst Review Team and participate in reviewing grant protocols focused on nursing investigations. Several nurses within PCS have Harvard University faculty appointments. Clinical nurses, as well as senior researchers, have the opportunity to seek funding for collaborative research activities through the Harvard Catalyst program.

Nursing Research Day

Each May, during Nurse Recognition Week at MGH, the Munn Center actively orchestrates Nursing Research Day. Planning for this event occurs over the year and embodies the work of the Munn Center committees. This event includes an interactive poster session, the annual Yvonne L. Munn Nursing Research Lecture, and the presentation of research awards. Nursing Research Day provides a forum for all nurses to network with other nurse researchers from MGH, as well as with national scholars. It is an opportunity to discuss developments in nursing knowledge, explore new ideas obtained from clinical investigations, and explore new ideas around advancing nursing practice through research and performance improvement. Information presented during this day offers nurses an opportunity to showcase their important work with other disciplines from across the MGH community.

Abstract submissions for the interactive poster session are open to all members of the PCS nursing community and to faculty nurse scientists appointed through the Munn Center. Classes on abstract development are held early in the year by the Munn Center and the librarian. All abstracts are reviewed and approved for dissemination by members of the Doctoral Forum. Accepted abstracts are published by the Munn Center in a *Book of Abstracts* for dissemination on Nursing Research Day. Articles on abstract development include the following:

- Russell, C. L., & Ponferrada, L. (2012). How to develop an outstanding conference research abstract. *Nephrology Nursing Journal, 39*(4), 307–342.

- Bliss, D. (2012). Writing a successful research abstract. *Journal of Wound, Ostomy & Continence Nursing, 39*(3), 244–247.

- Bingham, R., & O'Neal, D. (2013). Developing great abstracts and posters. *Nursing for Women's Health, 17*(2), 131–138. doi:10.1111/1751-486X.12021

- Writing competitive scientific and clinical abstracts: Tips for success. (2013). *Canadian Journal of Cardiovascular Nursing, 23*(1), 19–20.

When abstracts are accepted for dissemination, the authors then prepare the posters for viewing throughout the first floor of the MGH. A Poster Awards Committee, led by the Munn Center, reviews all posters and selects poster award winners in three categories: original research, EBP, and performance improvement.

Nursing Research Grand Rounds

In 2013, the Munn Center in coordination with PCS, introduced Nursing Research Grand Rounds on a quarterly basis to the MGH community. These hour-long sessions are open to the entire MGH community across disciplines and designed to share the results of nursing research investigations and clinical inquiry in a collaborative research environment. Clinical nurses, as well as nurse scientists, have an opportunity to discuss research findings and the overall impact of study results on patient care, future research, and knowledge development.

All presentations are videotaped and available on the Munn Center website for all to view. Announcements of the presentation dates and topics to be discussed are prepared by the Munn Center and disseminated to the entire MGH and PCS community through email and publication in *Caring Headlines*. Presentations are often delivered by nurses who have received Munn Awards and other funded research awards or grants. The success of these presentations to date speaks to the quality of the presentations, the unique perspective of nursing research around clinical problems impacting all disciplines, the interest of other disciplines in the results of nursing inquiry, and the visible contributions of nursing research to patient care and the scientific community.

The Partners Human Research Committee (IRB)

All nurses participating in research studies must complete the IRB's online educational program, Collaborative Institutional Training Initiative (CITI) (http://www.citiprogram.org), prior to beginning the study. The CITI program was developed by experts in the "IRB community" and consists of two basic courses in the protection of human research subjects for biomedical as well as for social/behavioral research. CITI also offers case-based refresher courses for continuing education. Members of the MGH research community are required to take the basic biomedical course. All research grant submissions must have IRB approval. All authors submitting a PI project must review and complete the Clinical Quality Improvement/Measurement Checklist to determine whether their human subjects research project requires review from the IRB.

Innovation in Care Delivery

The Munn Center works with the Center for Innovation in Care Delivery to participate in the evaluation of practice interventions on patient care outcomes. This includes identification of variables and measures as well as the development of surveys to collect and evaluate data and impact. In addition to exploring the impact of innovation on nurse and patient satisfaction, quality, cost, safety, and sustainability, Munn Center staff work with the Center for Innovation team to explore the relationship between and among the innovation bundle and the patient care delivery model, the PPM, and other organizational data. You can read a more complete discussion of innovation-related evaluation in Chapter 5, "Supporting Operational Effectiveness and Encouraging Research Through Innovation."

Collaborative Governance Evidence-Based Practice Committee

The Munn Center participates in the work of EBP by serving as consultant to the Collaborative Governance Evidence-Based Practice Committee. Work of the committee includes generating research grants (e.g., Health Resources and Services Administration [HRSA] funding) to promote the development, implementation, and evaluation of educational programs delivered by clinical nurse specialists to increase staff knowledge of EBP by facilitating and mentoring EBP studies through the Munn Center. In addition, the co-chairs of the EBP Collaborative Governance Committee attend quarterly Munn Team meetings and meet with Munn Staff to discuss strategies that can be used to promote EBP.

At MGH, evidence-based standards of practice guide decision-making and activities of the Department of Nursing. Chapter 4, "Using, Evaluating, and Integrating an Evidence-Based Practice," discusses useful strategies that can enhance the knowledge and skills needed by the workforce to examine current evidence and develop new evidence, generate opportunities for staff to engage in mentored EBP projects (e.g., Munn Awards) and support the translation and use of evidence into care delivery practice models.

Magnet Recognition Program®

In all the activities within the Munn Center, continuous attention is paid to developing, evaluating, and storing data to be utilized as sources of evidence for Magnet® recognition. All projects initiated have an evaluation component, and the evidence produced becomes part of evidence submitted to address specific Magnet Recognition Program® standards. The work of the Munn Center reflects visionary, transformative, leadership, creativity, and implementation of new approaches to care delivery and workforce development. From the generation of a team agenda to the development of the grant tracker, the Munn Center's initiatives have evolved as the requirements for Magnet recognition have evolved.

The development of new instruments to evaluate workforce satisfaction, the evaluation data to determine the effectiveness of innovation projects, and the evidence obtained from funded research all provide data that support Magnet Recognition Program standards and gives a new voice to nursing's impact on patient care. The Munn Center helps to actualize the PPM, and more importantly, it evaluates its impact over time. It contributes examples that reflect visionary thinking and evaluates the role of transformative leadership on creating a professional practice care environment (see Chapter 8, "Evaluating Professional Practice in Nursing Research"). The work of the Munn Center contributes evidence around the impact of nursing on care outcomes through research. Chapter 9, "The Magnet Recognition Program® Journey: An Engine for Research and Evidence-Based Practice," provides a complete discussion linking nursing research to Magnet recognition.

Clinical Research Nurses Roundtable

The clinical research nurse is actively involved in the implementation of approved research protocols at MGH. This group of research nurses participates in the implementation of clinical research investigations in patient care settings, or in clinical research units designed to support clinical research. The number of clinical research nurses at MGH is significant. In 2014, the group spearheaded an initiative that resulted in the MGH group becoming the first chapter in the newly formed International Association of Clinical Research Nurses (IACRN). The focus of the IACRN is to dialogue and set standards that impact their clinical nursing research activities. As the number of nurses securing grant funding that involves the implementation of clinical trials increases, an increased collaboration with the clinical research nurses may follow.

The MGH Clinical Research Center (CRC) continues to grow as the MGH research enterprise expands. The CRS provides support for nurse scientists involved in the conduct human subject research. The nurse director of the CRC is a member of the Munn quarterly team meeting and provides updates about opportunities for nurse scientists to obtain support for research from the center. The CRC at MGH is expanding, and it is expected that as more nurses are involved in clinical trials, the number of nursing protocols implemented by clinical research nurses will also increase. The Munn Center team meetings also include the co-chairs of the MGH Clinical Research Nurses Roundtable. It is anticipated that collaborations between this Munn Center and the clinical research nurses will be an important affiliation as nursing research expands.

Executive Committee on Research (ECOR) and the MGH Research Enterprise

The growth of research within the MGH and across Partners HealthCare is being realized in new initiatives that expand the development and translation of the research, increase the development of databases, and advance the infrastructure to store, retrieve, and analyze large data sets to improve care. The Executive Committee on Research (ECOR) at the MGH is focused on the development of this research enterprise that is working to extend the resources, data availability, education, and support for all researchers. Nurses from PCS and the Munn Center have become active participants in this project and are members of the committees identified within ECOR. The Munn Center is identified within the emerging organizational structure of ECOR and is part of research activities at the MGH. Nurses and nurse scientists within PCS participate in the Research Council and are on committees to promote collaborative research opportunities across disciplines. Doctorally prepared nurses are invited to share their research interests and expertise on a multidisciplinary website and they can be called upon by other scientists to join discussion across groups to promote clinical research investigations. The inclusion of nurse researchers in this initiative supports the visibility of nursing inquiry and discovery.

Partners Clinical Research Program

The Clinical Research Program (CRP) offers multiple educational programs and related support for scientists at all stages of the clinical research process. Nurse researchers can access programs and resources on the CRP website. The CRP provides a number of classes on research development and implementation essential for the conduct of clinical investigations. The director of the CRP serves on Munn Center committees, attends the quarterly Munn Center team meetings, and serves as a member of the Connell Nursing Research Scholars (CNRS) advisory group.

Grant Development and Submission

The staff at the Munn Center meets with nurses on a regular basis to facilitate grant development and submission, publication, and manuscript development and to provide mentoring and consultation. Munn Center staff work with nurse researchers to help interpret proposal guidelines, review and edit sections of a grant submissions, and develop a timeline for required documents to be submitted to the MGH Grants and Contracts Office. Projects submitted for funding extend the researcher's body of work and are expected to align with the strategic goals of the IPC and PCS.

Munn Center Grant Review Process

After staff researchers have identified a project and a grant mechanism they wish to apply to for funding, they are encouraged to meet with members of the Munn staff. To make these meetings more helpful, the staff researchers are asked to submit a concept paper prior to their initial meeting with the Munn Center team that covers the following outline:

Grant purpose: What institute/agency do you want a grant from? Briefly describe the purpose of the grant.

Problem/background: Explain why you think this topic needs a study. Demonstrate you know the institute's priorities.

Significance: Explain why this is important to the field of inquiry and discipline.

Question: What hypotheses will you test and what model will guide your hypotheses?

Design/methods/analysis: What is the study design that will enable testing your hypotheses? What is your statistical approach?

Team: Who will be the key participants (co-investigators and organizations) on the project?

Miscellaneous: Other relevant information.

Additional assistance with abstract development occurs at several times throughout the year. Classes offered through the Munn Center are available to all staff interested in submitting an abstract for a conference, grant submission, or MGH Research Day poster presentation or the MGH Clinical Research Day. (Refer to the resources listed in the "Nursing Research Day" section of this chapter.)

The CRP provides a variety of services to investigators around research methods. Statistical support is offered through both the CRP and Munn Center. The Munn Center provides assistance and consultation to nurse researchers in liaison with the MGH Office of Grants and Contracts, the office within Partners Research Administration. Budget preparation is offered through the Munn Center and the grant manager (GM). All MGH nurses interested in receiving grant consultation, complete the Research Consultation form and submit it to the Munn Center for follow up by Munn Center staff. The following sidebar offers examples of grant submission activities accomplished through the Munn Center.

EXAMPLE GRANT PREPARATION AND REVIEW PROCESS IN THE MUNN CENTER

Grant Submission/Consultation Service Guidelines

Munn Center nurse scientists and staff meet with nurses about perspective grant and research opportunities. Prior to meeting with the Munn staff, each staff member or researcher completes a consultation form that can be downloaded from the Munn Research website (www.mghpcs.org/MunnCenter). The form is then sent to the center, and an appointment date is arranged. Staff in the Munn Center review guidelines of proposed grants, review and edit proposals, and assist with submission timelines through the MGH Grants and Contracts Office.

Munn Center Grant Review Process

Applicants are asked to identify a topic, grant mechanism, and research focus. Initial and follow-up feedback is provided by a Munn Center review team. Completed grants are reviewed using an adapted version of the National Institutes of Health (NIH) grant review form.

Assistance Through the Clinical Research Program (CRP) & Statistical Support

The CRP provides a variety of services (including project consultation) to investigators for a variety of research methods. Statistical support is offered through the CRP as well as well as the Munn Center by appointment. The website for the CRP is http://www.massgeneral.org/crp/.

Assistance with Budget & Contracts for Submitted Grants

The Munn Center provides assistance and consultation to nurse researchers in liaison with the MGH Office of Grants and Contracts, the office within Partners Research Administration. All completed proposals are submitted directly from the Munn Center to the Office of Grants and Contracts and then by Grants and Contracts to the respective funding agency.

Since the dedication of the Munn Center within the Institute for Patient Care in 2008, MGH nurses have had the opportunity and guidance to design research projects and write research grant proposals to fund these projects. Programs of nursing research and interdisciplinary investigation in the Munn Center and across PCS are evolving. Currently, the focus is on a variety of research initiatives that complement the PCS's strategic agenda. Current areas of nursing research under exploration include the following:

- Care of the Older Adult and Palliative Care

- Workforce Evaluation

- Evaluation of the Professional Practice Model (PPM)

- Symptom Management (e.g., pain, skin breakdown/pressure ulcers, infection, falls)

- Complementary Healing Interventions

- Population-Based Care

- Impact/Outcome Educational Research

- Transitional Care

Between 2008 and 2114, MGH nurse researchers have submitted over 110 grant applications to intramural and extramural agencies and secured funding for 39 research projects. In addition, the Munn Center was awarded a significant funding from the William F. Connell Foundation to develop a Connell Nursing Research Scholars Program and a Connell Ethics Fellowship program. Table 3.3 provides examples of external grants funded.

TABLE 3.3 Examples of Internal and External Funded Grant Projects in the Munn Center

FUNDING SOURCE	GRANT TITLE
American Association of Retired Persons (AARP)	Age Wise: Care of the Elderly Training Program
Health Services Research Administration (HRSA)	Retooling for Evidence-Based Nursing Practice
External philanthropic funding	Connell Nursing Research Scholar Awards (for postdoctoral research development)

FUNDING SOURCE	GRANT TITLE
Occupational Safety and Health Administration (OSHA) NIOSH Award	The Feasibility and Efficacy of Using a Computer-Assisted Pedometer Aimed at Increasing Daily Steps Taken, Improving Mood, and Decreasing the Amount of Time Being Sedentary
Occupational Safety and Health Administration (OSHA) NIOSH Award	Exploring the Experience and Impact of Therapeutic Touch Treatments to Nurse Colleagues
Health Services Research Administration (HRSA)	Clinical Ethics Residency Training Program for Nurses
NIH/NINR R-15 Secondary Contract	Effects of a Nurse-Coached Intervention Following Same Day Arthroscopic Surgery
American Association of Colleges of Nursing (AACN)	MGH CICU Implements the ABCDE Bundle—Respiratory Care
Internal: Yvonne L. Munn Postdoctoral Fellowship in Nursing Research	Secondary Analysis of the Pain Assessment Instrument: Pain Assessment and Care for the Extremely Low Gestational Age Infant Focused Instrument (PACEFI) Data Set
Internal: Yvonne L. Munn Nursing Research Award Munn Award—Staff	Comparison of Temporal Artery to Pulmonary Artery Thermistor Temperatures in Hyperthermic Patients
Internal: Yvonne L. Munn Nursing Research Award Munn Award—Staff	Patients' Experiences of Hatha Yoga During Autologous Hematopoietic Stem Cell Transplant
Robert Wood Johnson Foundation INQRI	The Nursing Ambulatory to Hospital Transition Program

In addition, many nurses across PCS and the MGH community are involved in advancing nursing conceptualizations that link philosophical and disciplinary knowledge with patient- and family-centered care and cost-effective, high-quality, safe patient outcomes.

Policy Development

Multiple policies have been developed by the Munn Center staff to guide the development, implementation and evaluation of research. In addition, policies that impact the conduct and implementation of committee work have also been implemented. One example of a policy implemented by the Munn Center in 2015 involved student research experiences at MGH. The policy delineated that:

> *"All student research practicum experiences will be cleared through the Professional Development Coordinator in the Institute for Patient Care before involving staff and the Munn Center."*

The goal of this policy is to monitor the number of requests for research practica, monitor staff preceptor and patient burden, and attempt to control the number of requests for student research experiences. To accomplish this, the Student Research Practicum Experience Request form was developed, and all students seeking a research experience at MGH are asked to complete the form and have it reviewed by IPC staff before implementation of the research practicum. Essential components of the form include a signature from the MGH site preceptor as well as the student's research faculty advisor to ensure that the experience will be monitored by the faculty working with each student. The form also asks students to attest that that they are certified and able participate in the conduct of research at MGH.

Scholarship

The dissemination of nursing knowledge through publications and presentations by MGH scholars occurs at an international level. Multiple publications from nurse scientists and scholars across PCS have contributed significant knowledge to the literature. The following list provides a sample of the scholarship that demonstrates significant dissemination of research activities:

- Adams, J. M., Nikolaev, N., Ives Erickson, J., & Jones D. A. (2013). Development and psychometric evaluation of the leadership influence over professional practice environment scale. *Journal of Nursing Administration, 43*(5), 258–265.

- Adams, J. M. (2014). Guest editorial: How do we know if we're innovating? A strategy for innovation evaluation in a practice setting. *Journal of Nursing Administration, 44*(2), 63–64.

- Carroll, D. L., Dykes, P. C., & Hurley, A. H. (2010). Patients' perspectives of falling while in an acute care hospital and suggestions for prevention. *Applied Nursing Research, 23,* 238–241.

- Carroll, D. L., & Gonzalez, C. E. (2009). Visiting preferences of cardiovascular patients. *Progress in Cardiovascular Nursing, 24*(4), 159–154.

- Carroll, D. L. (2014). Factors influencing recovery for older adults and spouses after a cardiovascular procedure. *International Journal of Nursing Practice, 20,* 97–105.

- Erickson, J. I., Duffy, M. E., Ditomassi, M., & Jones, D. (2009, May). Psychometric evaluation of the Revised Professional Practice Environment (RPPE) scale. *Journal of Nursing Administration, 39*(5), 236–43.

- Flanagan, J., Winters, L. N., Habin, K., & Cashavelly, B. (2012). Women's experiences with antiestrogen therapy to treat breast cancer. *Oncology Nursing Forum, 39*(1), 70–77.

- Jones, D., Duffy, & M., Flanagan, J. (2011). A randomized clinical control trial testing the efficacy of a nurse-coached intervention (NCI) in arthroscopy patients. *Nursing Research, 60*(2), 92–99.

- Jones, D., Duffy, M. E., Flanagan, J., & Foster, F. (2012) Psychometric evaluation of the functional health pattern assessment screening tool (FHPAST). *International Journal of Nursing Knowledge, 23*(3), 140–145.

- Lee, S., Coakley, E., Dahlin, C., & Ford-Carleton, P. (2009). An evidence-based nurse residency program in geropalliative care. *Journal of Continuing Education in Nursing, 40*(12), 536–542.

- Looby, S. E. (2012). Menopause-associated metabolic manifestations and symptomatology in HIV Infection: A brief review with research implications. *Journal of the Association of Nurses in AIDS Care, 23*(3), 195–203.

- Looby, S. E., Shifren, J., Corless, I., Rope, A., Pedersen, M. C., Joffe, H., & Grinspoon, S. (2014). Increased hot flash severity and related interference in perimenopausal HIV-infected women. *Menopause: The Journal of the North American Menopause Society, 21*(4), 403–409.

- Perry, D. (2005). Transcendent pluralism and the influence of nursing testimony on environmental justice legislation. *Policy, Politics & Nursing Practice, 6*(1), 60–71.

- Stamp K. D., Flanagan, J., Gregas, M., & Shindul-Rothschild, J. (2014). Predictors of excess heart failure readmissions. *Journal of Nursing Care Quality, 29*(2), 115–123.

In addition, there have been a number of collaborations and partnerships within and across disciplines around instrument development and related research initiatives (qualitative and quantitative methods) used to support the psychometric evaluation of these tools. The following list provides a sample of these instruments:

- **Patient Care Assistant Workforce Environment Scale:** Developed in collaboration with Munn Center staff and PCS leadership

- **Staff Perceptions of the Professional Practice Environment Survey:** Developed in collaboration with Munn Center staff and PCS leadership

- **Disruptive Behavior in Workplace Scale:** Developed in collaboration with Munn Center staff, nursing, and the Department of Psychiatry staff (paper in review)

- **Effectiveness of Innovation Survey - Impact and Sustainability:** Developed in collaboration with Munn Center staff, the Center for Innovations in Care Delivery team, and PCS leadership

- **Adaptations of the Staff Perceptions of the Professional Practice Environment Survey for Orthopedic Surgical Group:** Developed for a cohort of staff across disciplines (e.g., the orthopedic surgeons, nurses, certified nurse anesthetist's (CRNAs) and anesthesiologists)

- **The MGH case managers (nursing) Staff Perception of the Professional Practice Environment Survey:** Developed for Case Managers within MGH

- **Requests for the Staff Perceptions of the Professional Practice Environment Tool Internationally (United States, Canada, China, Spain, and so on):** Specific request form on the Munn Center website.

For example, the evaluation of the professional practice addresses the impact of components of the PPE and how they correlate to better patient and organizational outcomes. The Revised Professional Practice Environment (RPPE) scale is intended to measure staff perceptions of eight components of the professional clinical practice environment in the acute care setting. Each subscale has been validated as a standalone measure, and together they provide a clear picture of staff perceptions of the environment in which they practice. The eight components of the RPPE, as well as other examples of research and instrument development, are discussed in Chapter 5.

Summary

The development of the Munn Center at the MGH continues to evolve. Since its inception in 2008, the Center has been a stimulus for inquiry and a support for staff interested in research and discovery. New opportunities to advance a nursing research agenda have been provided, with new opportunities for research available to doctorally prepared nurses. These developments have helped to create a culture of inquiry for all nurses. The research activities initiated by nurses continue to foster a nursing research agenda that generates new knowledge and innovations in practice that promote healing and relieves suffering.

The emerging research agenda realized through the work of the Munn Center has been communicated to the scientific community in high-impact journals and international presentations. This visibility has identified MGH as a leader in the advancement of nursing knowledge within a practice environment as evidenced by original research and EBP initiatives. Continued funding, expansion of research opportunities, development of nurse-led interdisciplinary research teams, and the influence of research outcomes that impact patient care continue to be realized. The growth of new partnerships and the expansion of multisite and international research investigations will increase knowledge development globally. In the end, the emergence of new investigations with evolving methodological approaches will advance nursing science and contribute knowledge that improves the health for all citizens of the world.

References

Duffy, M. (2013). Measuring the hospital work environment. In Ives Erickson, J., Ditomassi, M., & Jones, D. A. (2013) *Fostering care at the bedside: Professional practice for the bedside leader from Massachusetts General Hospital* (pp. 275-305). Indianapolis, IN: Sigma Theta Tau International.

Ives Erickson, J., Ditomassi, M., & Jones, D. A. (2013) *Fostering care at the bedside: Professional practice for the bedside leader from Massachusetts General Hospital.* Indianapolis, IN: Sigma Theta Tau International.

Jones, D. A. (2009). Yvonne L. Munn Center for Nursing Research (brochure). Boston, MA: MGH Press, 2.

Munn Center Nursing Research Award. (n.d.). Retrieved from http://www.mghpcs.org/MunnCenter/Munn_Center_Research_Award.asp

Chapter 4
Using, Evaluating, and Integrating an Evidence-Based Practice

–Diane L. Carroll, PhD, RN, FAAN

–Howard T. Blanchard, MEd, MS, RN, ACNS-BC, CEN

In recent years, a number of forces have created the momentum essential for nursing practice to be evidence based. Multiple publications by the Institute of Medicine (IOM), including *To Err Is Human: Building a Safer Health System* (IOM, 2000), *Crossing the Quality Chasm: A New Health System for the 21st Century* (IOM, 2001, p. 22), and *The Future of Nursing: Leading Change, Advancing Health* (IOM, 2010), have been an important stimulus for nurses and other healthcare providers to use research and related evidence to guide decisions about care delivery. According to the IOM, evidence-based practice (EBP) is designed to provide consistent, high-quality patient care through implementing the best scientific knowledge, thereby limiting practice variations and making care efficient and safe (IOM, 2001, p. 22).

In addition to the IOM report support of EBP, many hospitals continue to seek and or sustain Magnet® recognition. This designation, established by the American Nurses Credentialing Center (ANCC), bestows recognition on those qualified healthcare organizations for their high-quality patient care, nursing excellence, and innovation in professional nursing practice (Luzinski, 2011; Wolf, Triolo, & Ponte, 2008). Embedded in the criteria for Magnet recogntion is the hospital's commitment to creating a culture of evidenced-based nursing and intra-professional practice. Vital competencies for nurses include use of EBP as well as the research process to answer questions related to patient care (IOM, 2010).

This chapter focuses on clarifying terminology used to describe EBP. It also discusses the EBP model and the strategies used within Massachusetts General Hospital (MGH) to promote and translate the use of evidence in practice and describe the organizational structures and processes that help facilitate its implementation.

EBP Terminology

EBP is more than writing down a current practice, searching the web for three journal articles supporting your practice and citing them at the end of a docu-ment. While many EBP definitions are found in the literature, DiCenso, Cullum, and Ciliska (1998) describe EBP as a model for clinical decisions. But EBP can also be viewed from a conceptual perspective with contributing elements, from exploring examples of how nurses have implemented EBP in their practice, and from innovative approach, to the use of EBP in current nursing practice.

Accepting a useful definition of EBP has taken several decades to achieve (Green, Ottoson, Garcia, & Hiatt, 2009). In 1996, Sackett and colleagues (p. 71) stated that EBP medicine means:

> "*Integrating* individual clinical expertise *with the* best available external clinical evidence *from systematic research. By individual clinical expertise we mean the proficiency and judgment that individual clinicians acquire through clinical experience and clinical practice. Increased expertise is reflected in many ways, but especially in more effective and efficient diag-nosis and in the more thoughtful identification and compassionate use of individual patients' predicaments, rights, and preferences in making clini-cal decisions about their care.*"

The three key concepts related to definitions of EBP (patient, evidence, and expertise) were articulated and developed over time, and are evident in earlier publications by Oxman, Sackett, and Guyatt (1993). This conceptualization reflects the importance of EBP as a process that involves more than translating research results into practice using clinical experience. Rather, EBP requires knowledge of individual patient information elicited through a careful history, physical examination, and other investigations. Clarity around the definition of EBP, as noted, is important to fully address a nurse-centric approach to EBP. These components, in addition to the three components of EBP medicine (research evidence, clinical expertise, and patient preferences), provide a more comprehensive definition of multiple elements important to EBP, as noted in Figure 4.1.

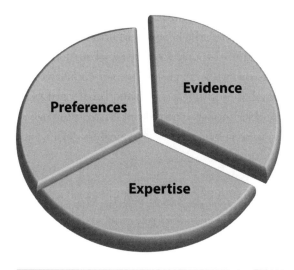

FIGURE 4.1

The Key Concepts of Evidence-Based Practice
Source: Original work by author: Howard T. Blanchard

Though the word *evidence* appears prominently in EBP, the entirety of the success in improving patient outcomes using EBP also includes clinical expertise and patient preferences. Each of the three components are weighted equally.

These key concepts have been reaffirmed by the IOM in their charter on Value and Science-Driven Health Care, which states that by 2020 learning health systems must achieve the following (Alston et al., 2012, p.1):

> *"90 percent of clinical decisions will be supported by accurate, timely, and up-to-date clinical information and will reflect the best available evidence. A continuously learning health system can deliver truly patient-centered care only when patient preferences, informed by medical evidence and provider expertise, are elicited, integrated, and honored."*

EBP Focus

Evidence, as a word or concept, is not the focus of EBP, or the goal of EBP. The focus of EBP is the patient, the nurse, and their health outcomes. Research, and the peer-reviewed evidence it provides, is made relevant through the processes performance quality improvement, research utilization, and scientific inquiry and the access of knowledge through research. The processes, such as research utilization, are led by clinically expert staff nurses and clinical nurse specialists at the point of care. The goal is to assist patients in reaching their goals safely and with quality outcomes, utilizing healthcare resources, improving health outcomes, decreasing overall costs, and generally increasing satisfaction with healthcare (Keele, 2011; Titler, 2008; Titler et al., 2001; Webb, 2011).

Performance/Quality Improvement

Performance or quality improvement consists of systematic and continuous actions that lead to measurable improvement in healthcare services and the health status of targeted patient groups (HSRA, 2011). Quality improvement work is evidence based as it is grounded in the common nature of being quantitative and iterative. These projects require a review of the goal of the work, defining of the selected patient group, what knowledge will be gained, and the burdens placed on the healthcare service (Newhouse & Pettit, 2006).

Research Utilization

Research utilization is the critical "examination and application of research findings to solve a clinical practice problem" (Keele, 2011; Titler, 2008). This examination and application of research are inclusive of all aspects of the nursing process and EBP. Research utilization includes nurses at all levels, and is applied at the point of caring for a patient problem. Using incremental processes of care improvement, research utilization coalesces these steps to ensure the achievement of optimum patient outcomes. In a five-hospital system on the East Coast of the United States, nurses described variability in their awareness of research utilization. This variability was based on a nurse's position within an organization, and their educational level, with advanced practice nurses more engaged in research utilization when compared to staff nurses (McClosky, 2008).

Research means a systematic investigation, including development, testing, and evaluation, designed to advance or contribute to generalizable knowledge (Department of Health and Human Services, 2009). Scholarly activities conducted or supported under a program that meets this definition may be considered research.

Nursing research is the exacting science that seeks to generate new knowledge, or is clarifying or confirming existing knowledge, to answer questions relevant to nursing practice (Titler, 2008; Webb, 2011). Nursing research is also the actual participation or conduct of empirical research studies (Keele, 2011). It is a separate and distinct area from EBP, and research utilization, though it is both informed by and informs EBP.

The EBP Implementation Model

The conceptual understanding and implementation of EBP at Massachusetts General Hospital (MGH), Patient Care Services (PCS), was fostered by a grant funded by the Division of Nursing, the Bureau of Health Professions, the Health Resources and Services Administration, and the Department of Health and Human Services Administration under D11HPO14632, Retooling for Evidence-Based Nursing Practice (Lee & Brandt, 2013). This project resulted in a model that affirmed the work of medicine to include an EBP model that combined the work of others in EBP medicine and redefining and applying principles and concepts of EBP to integrate nursing and the three key aspects of EBP: research evidence, clinical expertise, and patient preference (Sackett, Rosenberg, Muir Gray, Harnes, & Richardson, 1996).

After careful consideration, the model selected to guide the EBP initiative was the Iowa Model of Evidence-Based Practice to Promote Quality Care (Titler et al., 2001). This model uses a decision tree to support healthcare professionals' recognition of when a decision point is reached and when it is necessary to review evidence available to guide the change, make the best choices to advance the practice, pilot proposed practice changes, and follow up (evaluate) to determine if the outcomes improved in practice (Titler et al., 2001). In later writing on the Iowa Model of Evidence-Based Practice to Promote Quality Care, Titler (2008) describes EBP as "the conscientious and judicious use of current best evidence in conjunction with clinical expertise and patient values to guide health care decisions" (Titler, 2008). At MGH and within PCS, EPB continues to be common practice. In addition, when various options for care exist, and available evidence is available to inform choices and subsequent actions, the patient is ultimately the person central to the final decision.

EBP Components

Several elements are of critical importance to the implementation and use of EBP at the MGH. They include patient preferences and values, and clinical nursing expertise, including knowledge, inquiry, and pattern identification. This focus enhances a patient/family-centric focus within the context of nurse-patient relationship-based care.

Evidence and EBP

Evidence is a distracting word within EBP. Focused as we are on clinical evidence as a part of EBP, it is integral but no more significant than clinical expertise and patient values. The current best evidence is evaluated by using tools such as LEGEND (Let Evidence Guide Every New Decision) of Cincinnati Children's

Hospital, with their copyrighted materials available on their website (James M. Anderson Center for Health Systems Excellence, 2014). This is one of the numerous taxonomies in use for rating nursing evidence. The Agency for Healthcare Research and Quality's Evidence Report/Technology Assessment Number 47 (2002) describes a number of scales, checklists, and rating systems at our disposal to evaluate evidence.

MORE ABOUT LEGEND

The Cincinnati Children's Hospital developed LEGEND (Let Evidence Guide New Decision) to assist in evaluations of evidence to determine impact on patient outcomes. LEGEND is a set of evidence evaluation tools and resources to guide evidence-based decision-making. The tools on its website (http://www. cincinnatichildrens.org/service/j/anderson-center/evidence-based-care/legend/) are:

- *Evaluating the evidence algorithm resource*

- *Evidence appraisal forms*

- *Tables of evidence levels*

- *Grading evidence tools*

- *Tools to judge the strength of a recommendation*

The tools are in a PDF format that are easily found on a two-axis grid on this website. Specifically, the grid addresses the research question asked, and the type of research design being evaluated. These forms are able to be used by nurses with little experience in rating evidence, and are effective on grading evidence for reviews.

Sackett and colleagues (1996) noted that the "best available external clinical evidence" is used in EBP (p. 71). The proliferation of published information creates challenges in identifying the best available evidence. The National Guideline Clearinghouse, Agency for Healthcare Research and Quality (AHRQ), U.S. Department of Health & Human Service provides evidence-based clinical practice guidelines. Other evidence-based resources such as the Cochrane Database of Systematic Reviews provide peer-reviewed systematic reviews or other expert evaluation features. At MGH, medical librarians are available to assist in developing search strategies for databases, including CINAHL and MEDLINE, and providing journal article links. In addition, the gray literature that encompasses a wide range of resources, including dissertations and reports, is available but requires skills to critically evaluation these information resources.

Evidence can be elusive, not because the subject has not been studied, but by the nature of the steps in the publication process. The partiality of journals to publish positive findings creates a bias to what we have to examine (Kark, 2012). Fortunately, negative findings are published. For example, presentation of an informational video to patients about to undergo a cardiac catheterization has been shown to improve satisfaction over a group who received the standard of care. Though the use of an informational video for patients about to undergo a cardiac catheterization demonstrated no reduction in anxiety state, the publication of this study saves other researchers from unknowingly retesting similar hypotheses (Gavigan, Cain, & Carroll, 2014).

EBP can occur only when all three key components are incorporated into healthcare decisions. Melnyk, Fineout-Overholt, Stillwell, and Williamson (2011) suggest that the influence afforded patient preference, clinical expertise, or the research evidence changes given the particular set of circumstances. Acute life or limb-saving actions are more prescribed than at the contrary end of a spectrum on the road of a patient's health continuum. EBP can be seen in an empowered patient that is participatory in seeking and choosing healthcare, and supported by expert clinicians who are able to share a comprehensive understanding of the current existing research-based information to inform healthcare decisions.

Patient Values and Preferences

Though *evidence* is a key word in EBP, the purpose behind EBP is patient-focused care and attaining the outcomes that are important to patients and their families. The second provision of the *Code of Ethics for Nurses* reads, "The nurse's primary commitment is to the patient, whether an individual, family, group, or community" (ANA, 2010a, p. 11). The interpretive statements are clear in stipulating that the patient has rights as a participant in the healthcare decision-making process and formulation of the care plan. Ethical issues, in particular, are resolved with a clear understanding of three things:

- The healthcare circumstances

- Those persons involved

- The patient's values and wishes

Within the framework of relationship-based care at MGH, personalized care planning is the form of shared decision-making (Coulter, 2012). The extent to which a nurse knows the patient and family can assist in developing a patient-specific plan of care. This patient knowledge aspect is vital to EBP. A plan can be viewed from various perspectives, including patient goals and what is meaningful to them and their decisions, culture, as well as the genome, or risk perspective.

"Cultural competence is represented as a quantifiable set of individual attitudes and communication and practice skills that enables the nurse to work effectively within the cultural context of individuals and families from diverse backgrounds" (Gustafson, 2005, p.2). For example, a patient from Asia was transferred to MGH for care. The healthcare providers from the outside hospital expressed concern about the patient's safety and autonomy within the home environment. Their rationale for this concern was a combination of observed family interactions with a patient who appeared passive, the hovering daughter, and the son who appeared to be the ultimate decision-maker. Shortly after the patient's arrival on the unit and the staff's understanding of the patient's culture and family relationship, viewed as culturally appropriate during a family illness, the staff was able to move beyond suspicion to engaging in care that was productive, responsive, and supportive for the family-as-patient (Nowak, 2005).

Other examples of a patient preference can differ from the research, evidence, and informed clinical choice of providers due to the patient or family perception that the treatment proposed is a risk or threat to the individual. Devereaux et al. (2001) studied patient versus physician decisions regarding the use of a drug (warfarin) as an antithrombotic treatment intervention. These researchers reported how evaluating the risk-benefits of a treatment influenced patient's decision-making. Study findings reported that patients indicated a greater readiness to accept a treatment (in this instance, an elevated possibility of bleeding on warfarin) to achieve a decrease risk of experiencing a stroke. MacLean and colleagues' (2012) analysis of 48 studies also concluded that patients can have varied preferences with respect to their thromboprophylaxis treatment choices. The researchers recommended that a discussion of patient preferences be part of clinical guidelines. Knowing the patient and coming to understand personal meanings associated with important choices and decisions reflect a valuing of patients and their participation in decisions and choices linked to their care. The focus on relationship-based care at MGH promotes strategies that can be used by the nurse and other providers to come to know patients and their goals of care.

Provision One of the ANA *Code of Ethics* entrusts nurses with respect for the inherent dignity of the patient (ANA, 2010a, p.1). The interpretation of this provision challenges nurses to know the patient well enough to accurately advance the patient's complete autonomy of choice. Provision Eight holds nursing responsible for understanding and meeting the ethnic and culturally diverse needs of our patients (ANA, 2010a, p. 103).

Clinical Nursing Expertise

Knowledge, inquiry, and pattern identification comprise the second component critical to linking empirical evidence and patient-focused care. Early in nursing evolution of EBP work, clinical expertise became the crucial element that separated evidence-based nursing from tradition-based care (DiCenso et al., 1998). Using Benner's narrative approach to patient care, the proficient nurse offers nursing care that utilizes effective clinical reasoning in a dynamic setting to synchronize care delivery practice with patient responses to the situation. The nurse is aware of change and has the ability to distinguish significance. "Expert practice is characterized by increased intuitive links between seeing the salient issues in a situation and ways of responding to them" (Benner, Tanner, & Chesla, 2009, p. 137).

Knowledge and EBP

Nursing continues to support increased educational preparation as critical to entry into nursing practice. Researchers have demonstrated an important link between improved patient outcomes and the educational nurse preparation of nursing (Aiken, Clarke, Cheung, Sloane, & Silber, 2003). These authors noted that a 'logical (but unconfirmed) connection between education and clinical judgment' (Aiken et al., 2003, p. 8).

Provision Five of the ANA *Code of Ethics* addresses the moral responsibility to self (as a nurse) and others (patients) to maintain competence and to continue personal and professional growth (ANA, 2010a). While accrediting bodies determine the minimum educational required to sit for the RN nursing licensure exam, continued review of the knowledge is necessary to ensure the expertise needed to meet an ever-evolving level of competency. Recommendations within the IOM report on *The Future of Nursing: Leading Change, Advancing Health* (IOM, 2010) promote nurses' participation in lifelong learning experiences to ensure that nurses have the knowledge and skills essential to offer culturally competent care throughout a patient's lifetime. In addition, this same IOM report supports the educational goal for the nursing workforce to consist of at least 80% baccalaureate nurses by 2020 in an effort to facilitate the complexity in the current healthcare environment.

McHugh and Lake (2010) cite Benner's (1984) work when they state "clinical expertise is a hybrid of practical and theoretical knowledge." Work by researchers at the University of Pennsylvania recognized the distinct concepts, education and experience, and what these concepts have added to defining expertise (Aiken et al., 2003; Kutney-Lee, Sloane & Aiken, 2013). These researchers reported a correlation of years of nursing experience and reported expertise as a "weak but statistically significant association" of highest education degree attained and their level of reported expertise, and the background effect of hospitals (McHugh & Lake, 2010). Hospitals with a higher percentage of baccalaureate-prepared nurses have an increased perception of clinical expertise (McHugh & Lake, 2010).

Inquiry, Technology, and Professional Development

There are two views regarding education:

- Formal education to an advanced degree

- Education within a nursing specialty by continuing education

In addition to the IOM's Report on the future of nursing (2010), which supports lifelong learning for nurses, Lenburg (2011) places professional development under the heading of both a professional and personal responsibility. Evolving clinical knowledge and innovations in technology challenge today's nurses. The use of new technologies to enhance nursing education and optimize patient care is changing and growing in importance. Each time we search the Internet for information, use a computer program to acquire new knowledge, interface with technology when caring for our patients, and communicate nursing care through electronic documentation (Lenburg, 2011), we are engaging in information exchange provided by technology. At MGH, for example, nurses are documenting electronically, replacing overhead paging with a text messages, and forwarding phone calls or updates directly to providers via smartphones. Patient education and the use of technology in the delivery of continuing education programs and simulation are additional examples of technology's impact on healthcare overall.

The ANA's *Code of Ethics* (2010) acknowledges that the ethics of professional growth and maintenance of competence is for the benefit of the patient, not for the nurse or the profession. Expert clinical knowledge and the use of clinical evidence, based on the patient's evolving condition, is how an expert clinician interacts with a particular patient condition to maximize the outcome (Benner et al., 2009).

Pattern Identification

Notice and *noticing* has entered the nursing vernacular to describe the initial insight the nurse has to stability or change in the patient response to an aspect of care. Watson and Rebair (2014) merged concepts from their earlier work on noticing to advance three conditions required for the nurse to notice:

- Experiential knowledge from clinical examples

- Educational learning, including textbooks

- Understanding of the particular patient's patterns

This knowledge is both supportive and reinforces the aspects of clinical nursing expertise as the basis for skilled care.

EPB and Clinical Nursing Expertise Example

The work of a clinically expert nurse, knowing and utilizing patient preferences within an environment, typically not malleable, to reach patient-expected outcomes is displayed in this example of clinical expertise.

The issue: I was part of the primary nurse team to care for K, a 41-year-old African-American woman, admitted with amyloidosis induced heart failure in need of a heart transplant. During her workup, the team discovered that K had multiple blood antibodies, blood type of O+, and an average size. This made the team realize that she could have a long wait for a donor heart, but we could not have predicted that her wait would be a year.

Clinical nurse specialist expertise: Assessment and knowing the person. K had an infectious smile and a good sense of humor. She had some idiosyncrasies and very high expectations of the staff. K orchestrated rounds each morning, allowing only the attending heart failure doctor to examine her. And the doctors were not welcome until after she had bathed. She also disliked white sheets. The nurse team used a blue lift pad on her bed to cover the white fitted bottom sheet, and her family brought in colored pillowcases.

K had to deal with many issues while hospitalized. There was isolation from family and friends and parenting long distance. She stayed connected with them through social media, by email, and by phone. Prior to hospitalization, K and her family often ate at fast-food restaurants. K said she liked to cook, but eating out seemed to be the norm. The unit nutritionist educated K regarding her diet and the importance of nutritious foods and a healthful diet. Staff were concerned K would slip back into bad habits once she returned home. Aggressive diuresis and dietary restrictions brought her weight down. She looked fabulous!

There is so much uncertainty surrounding a patient awaiting a transplant. As time went by, the wait became more and more difficult for K. Many doctors were involved in her care. Information about her status on the list and her antibodies was relayed to her through many different physicians. These frequent changes proved to be a challenge for her. She grew frustrated and angry when she received different answers to the same questions. The primary nurse team resolved this by assigning one doctor to answer her questions, and this proved very helpful.

The evidence-based outcome and expertise: K's primary nurse team developed strategies to help during her long wait for transplant. K had a strong faith. Staff provided her time each morning to pray and read her Bible. She kept a journal for writing down her thoughts. We took her to the hospital chapel and healing garden. Weather permitting, we would take K outside to enjoy the warm weather. We visited the hospital salon so that she could get her hair washed. She hated hospital gowns and robes, so family sent her own clothes from home. She said getting out of hospital clothes made her feel more human. The team would bring her laundry home to wash.

There are out-of-pocket expenses for patients waiting for a transplant, especially for patients from out of town. In K's case, the transplant social work contributed to accommodations for family along with bus tickets so that they could visit. For diversion, nurses contributed money so that a nurse could buy some lottery tickets. The tickets were attached to a board and presented to K. She spent an entire morning scratching tickets and won $150.

K's primary nurse team, along with our clinical nurse specialist, realized that her liberal diet could not continue post-transplant. We met with the clinical nurse specialists from the cardiac surgical unit and psychiatry. The primary nurse team told them a bit about K and the strategies they used to support K in hospital until her transplant. We then met with K and explained the need for her to follow her special diet more closely and that she would need to start to choose foods more carefully from the hospital menu. We made these changes gradually. K did complain, but her team responded with the same explanation and a united front. People have said the primary nurse team caring for K got her to transplant; without us, she would have gone home. We used atypical strategies to keep her healthy physically and mentally. I guess I agree with that, but I think that's what we do; we know our patients and use our combined clinical expertise to help our patients reach their goals.

Strategies to Promote and Translate Clinical Evidence

The chief nursing officer (CNO) and senior nursing leadership play a pivotal role in building the capacity for EBP. Defining and implementing an infrastructure that builds and sustains the capacity for EBP has accomplished a shift from nursing care steeped in tradition to a nursing culture that reflects on practice, seeks answers from the evidence, and applies these answers to patient care. When answers are not available, nurses use the research process to generate and disseminate new knowledge (Newhouse, 2007; Titler et al., 2001).

The CNO and senior nursing leadership implemented a number of promotional and translational strategies to sustain the organizational culture of EBP. This included collaborative governance with nurse-sensitive outcome subcommittees, a research and EBP committee, EBP orientation and continuing education, recognition, the role of the clinical nurse specialist (CNS), and the impact of the electronic medical record in EBP.

Collaborative Governance and EBP

Development of structures that encourage nursing's and other disciplines' responsibility for engaging in EBP initiatives is critical to promoting an EBP environment. At MGH, nurses can be part of a committee within collaborative governance (CG). The Evidence-Based Practice Committee's charge is to develop knowledge needed about EBP and to engage in activities that champion the development, use, and translation of evidence into practice. In conjunction with the CNSs, many frontline clinicians develop EBP projects at the unit level and work with the Yvonne L. Munn Center for Nursing Research (Munn Center) to present the findings to the community.

Encouraging nurses to be reflective in their practice includes questioning and seeking evidence to support the care they provide to patients. One of the components of the Magnet® Model is the requirement that nurses create new knowledge, care innovations, and care improvements. This refers to the belief that nurses have a professional responsibility to generate knowledge, implement innovation, know patient preferences, and focus on quality and safe patient care. Magnet-recognized organizations, such as MGH, design an infrastructure so that nurses can implement new models of care, ensure that nursing practice is evidence-based, and engage nurses as needed in the research process (ANCC, 2014).

Collaborative governance (CG) is the nursing and PCS communication and decision-making infrastructure at MGH. The CG structure is based on the belief that nurses own their practice and have a responsibility for advancing the science of nursing (Porter-O'Grady, 2001). The CG committee structure at MGH allows for the accountability and responsibility for making practice decisions that are guided by evidence to be in the hands of the clinicians who are the leaders at the bedside. Clinicians who participate in CG bring ideas, thoughts, and questions to the committees; communicate discussions and outcomes to their peers; and educate the organization.

Nurse-Sensitive Outcome Committees

According the American Nurses Association's *Nursing Scope and Standards of Practice* (ANA, 2010b), nurses are required to engage in self-evaluation of practice to ensure that current and best evidence is used to direct care. The formal structure for evaluating existing nursing practice is CG. In this model, a combination of practice and quality committees form the Collaborative Governance Practice and Quality Oversight Committee. The purpose of this committee is to ensure that an environment is created where patients received safe, evidence-based quality care delivered by competent clinicians.

At MGH, the Collaborative Governance Practice and Quality Oversight Committee oversees the work of five interdisciplinary subcommittees: Policy, Procedures, and Products; Pain Management; Skin Care; Fall Prevention; and the Restraint Usage. The clinician members of these subcommittees are the experts regarding practice, know the EBP for nursing interventions for these nurse-sensitive outcomes, and are the communicators of issues, interventions, and outcomes for the work of these committees to the organization.

The Policy, Procedures, and Products Subcommittee is responsible for reviewing and approving products, policies, and procedures to ensure that outcomes of their work is evidence based. Approved products that are brought into the practice environment must have an agreed upon rollout, with planned education and skills training as needed. The products may require a revision or a new policy and procedure to be developed to support the practice. The members of this subcommittee lead pilot trials of new products or processes in the clinical environment to inform this subcommittee.

The standard timeframe for review of current policies and procedures is every 3 years to ensure that all practice is based on current, up-to-date evidence and to review current research findings. The subcommittee uses organizational experts and known patient preferences in the review process. Using a systematic review, Restrepo, Jameson, and Carroll (2015) identified a need to revise the current procedure for mechanical prophylaxis for deep vein thrombosis. Based on the synthesis of the evidence, the policy now recommends the use of intermittent compression devices for the surgical patient instead of graduated compression stockings.

Nurse-Sensitive Outcomes and EBP Subcommittees

In an effort to increase the focus on critical areas of importance to patient care and related outcomes, a number of subcommittees were formed to address key patient care challenges, as follows:

- **The Pain Management Subcommittee:** The purpose of this subcommittee is to ensure that clinicians have the knowledge and skill to assess and treat patients' pain using the best evidence. The clinicians who serve on this committee are resources to the organization as they strive to improve patient satisfaction related to pain management. The committee members standardized the organizational approach to pain assessment through a comprehensive review of the evidence to identify the most valid and reliable age-appropriate and ability-appropriate pain assessments. These pain assessments were disseminated along with a list of resources for clinicians to use for assistance with assessment and pain management throughout the organization.

- **The Skin Care Subcommittee:** This subcommittee focuses their work on maintenance of skin integrity and prevention and treatment of acquired pressure ulcers. The committee members focus on the development of standard approaches to assessment of skin and treatment of altered skin integrity that reflect the current state of the science, the use of guidelines, and the evaluation of products that support the current clinical practice. The members of this subcommittee are the unit experts and resource for prevention and treatment of pressure ulcers. The subcommittee reviews organizational data to problem solve issues of altered skin integrity.

- **The Fall Prevention Subcommittee:** This subcommittee is charged with providing a safe environment for all patients and to develop individualized plans of care for patients who are at risk for falls. The subcommittee members use current evidence to develop a fall risk assessment and a comprehensive plan of care for fall prevention and to provide the organization with clear and current guidelines. With the use of the standard fall risk assessment, the Morse Falls Scale (Morse, 2008), the subcommittee utilized the research of Partners HealthCare colleagues to integrate the Morse Falls Scale into a fall prevention plan of care that is based on the patient's individualized risks for falls and evidence for appropriate nursing interventions (Dykes et al., 2010).

  The committee also reviews specific fall cases and the organizational fall rate data. The information that is gathered in the subcommittee has led to the development of post-fall unit-based discussions. These discussions include the clinicians and experts to foster not only unit-based evaluations but to also allow for organizational learning. Each patient fall requires a safety report that is used as a learning opportunity from the bedside clinician up to the board of trustees.

- **The Restraint Usage Subcommittee:** This subcommittee is engaged in identifying evidence-based interventions that can reduce the use of restraints. The subcommittee educates and teaches clinicians the skills they need to assess their patients and identify, based on patient risk, the most appropriate interventions that have evidence to support alternatives to restraints.

The subcommittee uses and reviews organizational data to develop performance improvement projects that utilize alternatives for restraints.

The committee members discussed the problems with using restraints and identified the need for seeking alternative solutions. The committee used expert opinion and expertise of clinicians who were part of the committee to seek a solution. The committee consulted with other institutions that had reduced their restraint use rates. One effective product identified was the protective arm sleeves. These sleeves protect intravenous access devices in those patients who, due to cognitive impairment, pull at intravenous devices. The committee reviewed the evidence on this as a method to reduce restraint usage and consulted with system-wide experts. The Restraint Usage Subcommittee designed two sequential trials to vet the protective arm sleeve with patients and staff to assess efficacy, comfort, and satisfaction. With data, the subcommittee proposed adoption of this product within the practice environment.

Research and Evidence-Based Practice Committee

The mission of the Research and Evidenced-Based Practice Committee is to welcome, reward, and disseminate new knowledge derived from clinical research and to support clinicians in the implementation of EBP. The committee membership is by application and consists of professionals from Speech and Language Pathology, Nursing, Social Service, and a medical librarian. Members are from diverse areas in the hospital.

In an effort to engage members of the committee within a culture of inquiry in a meaningful way, a portion of the meeting time is devoted to identifying research questions and to improving the ability of the members to search for and critique published evidence. Using a model to develop competencies in clinical inquiry, the goals of this committee were to have all clinicians literate with respect to the EBP components and skills (Stanley, Sitterding, Broome, & McCaskey, 2011) (see Figure 4.2). Annually, the librarian shares search techniques of organizational-supported databases. There were many critique tools discovered in the literature. After a review, the committee chose the evidence evaluation tools from the Cincinnati Children's Hospital, Let Evidence Guide Every New Decision (LEGEND), as the appraisal forms for grading evidence (Clark, Burkett, & Stanko-Lopp, 2009).

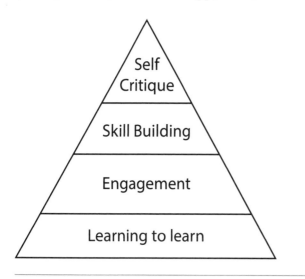

FIGURE 4.2

Pyramid of Learning for Competence in Clinical Inquiry
Educational processes and competencies developed by the
EBP team members over time.
Source: Stanley et al., 2011. Permission to reprint from Elsevier

The work on literacy for EBP was accomplished by sharing research examples with different levels of evidence and use of the LEGEND tools to evaluate and grade the evidence (James M. Anderson Center for Health Systems Excellence, 2014). The committee works in partnership with other CG committees to share evidence evaluation skills and to learn clinical content. The committee invites clinicians to participate in a critique of research that is pertinent to the content of the various subcommittees. For example, the Pain Management Subcommittee leadership brought pain assessment instruments to a meeting for review, critique, and discussion.

The clinicians of the committee use two activities to disseminate research that support EBP:

- **A summary of evidence poster on a specific topic:** The Did You Know posters are developed to share clinically pertinent topics using an evidence-based approach (see Chapter 9, "The Magnet Recognition Progam® Journey: An Engine for Research and Evidence-Based Practice"). The subcommittee clinicians work with content experts and medical librarians to produce posters that are distributed to all patient care units for clinician review. Examples of posters over the past year have been on skin assessment and on the appropriated use of the temporal artery thermometer, a standard at MGH.

- **An organizational-wide journal club:** The journal club, More Than Just a Journal Club, expanded the format for presentations to utilize the resources and experience of more researchers in the community and to partner with care units to co-host these researchers. For each presentation, the subcommittee members seek out researchers who are in the organization or the area and ask that they present their research article to the participants. Matching the research presentation to a specific unit that cares for the patients who are subjects in the research article increases the relevance to the participants. This has been a very successful strategy to put research findings in the hands of the clinician.

Nurse Orientation and Continuing Education

At MGH, the first day of nursing orientation contains a 50-minute lecture on EBP to initiate the new MGH nurse to the EBP culture. Opening with an inquiry regarding the range of backgrounds of the nurses attending, it is typical to discover a few returning nurses, as well as near 50% newly licensed nurses. The class, designed during the HRSA grant, Retooling for Evidence-Based Nursing Practice (Lee & Brandt, 2013), reaches approximately 270 new nurses each year. The lecture format, supported by a PowerPoint presentation, is energized by examples from practice and audience participation. Beginning with the EBP definition from Titler (2008), the discussion incorporates the three components of evidence, clinical expertise, and patient values. The new MGH nurse is presented examples of how every part is both critical and interdependent in reaching the goals of EBP.

After the initial orientation to EBP, the Norman Knight Nursing Center for Clinical and Professional Development offers specialized continuing education for PCS. This department develops courses that equate to 642 contact hours per year. Many of the continuing education offerings support the ongoing clinical knowledge requirements of the nurse in the current complex healthcare environment.

Recognition

In the mid-1990s, the CNO and senior nursing leadership instituted annual research/EBP awards. The purpose of these awards is to support staff nurses in their pursuit of nursing knowledge and improving health outcomes for patients. The intent is that these projects support and advance PCS goals and the professional practice of the nurse. Each year, during Nurse Recognition Week, a day is focused on EBP and research. The goal of this day is to recognize the contributions of nursing to the use of or development of nursing knowledge. There is an annual call for abstracts, an abstract review process, and support within PCS for the development of EBP and research posters. For 2 weeks, these posters are displayed in the main corridor of MGH for the hospital community, patients, and their families to view. See Table 4.1 for an example. These opportunities build and sustain a culture to support EBP.

TABLE 4.1 Current Evidence-Based Projects in Patient Care Services

Project title:
Digital air leak assessment after pulmonary resection: An observational study
Rechallenge after Paclitaxel-related infusion reactions in an oncology unit
A glimpse into the delicate dance that is the art of nursing

A multidisciplinary approach to improving nutritional status of patients at risk for pressure ulcers

A multidisciplinary collaboration to improve the care of high acuity patients on the inpatient psychiatric unit

Assessment of environmental modifications in family violence screening in the newborn intensive care unit

Glycemic control in the surgical intensive care unit with an insulin protocol

The use of a nasal brindle for naso-enteral tube feeding retention in the surgical intensive care unit

Head-to-toe, way to go! Skin assessment

Redesigning the Patient Observer Model to achieve increased efficiency and staff satisfaction

Using research to change practice in the Endoscopy Unit: Demerol versus Fentanyl for procedural sedation

Morphine first initiative

EPB and Use of Evidence Example

The issue: With a concern over the rising incidence of ventilator-associated pneumonia (VAP), the organization looked into the implementation of an EBP intervention for the prevention of VAP. The Institute for Healthcare Improvement developed a set of recommendations found to be very effective for the intubated patient at reducing VAP. The Ventilator Bundle, as the guideline was called, included a sequence of interventions linked to ventilator care and shown to significantly improve outcomes when implemented together, moreso than when they are implemented individually (Marra et al., 2009; Munro, Grap, Jones, McClish, & Sessler, 2009).

Current practice: The importance of proper oral care in patients, particularly for intubated individuals, is not a recent notion (Jenkins, 1986; Nesley, 1986). Current critical-care nursing manuals, as well as protocols issued by the

American Association of Critical-Care Nurses, advocate proper oral care using swabbing, tooth brushing, and suctioning of oral secretions (AACN, 2011). Despite the knowledge contained in these clinical sources on effective measures to reduce colonization in the oropharynx, the implementation of coordinated plans that include evidence-based interventions is not a common practice.

The EBP initiative: With an assessment of oral care interventions being used at MGH, it was acknowledged that within the organization, components of the oral care intervention were being completed but that the practice was inconsistent and variable. Units were using different products, and the frequency of oral care was unpredictable. Armed with this information, a task force of advanced practice nurses, staff, and quality nurses collected the evidence, reviewed the products that were available, and then trialed and evaluated various products from different vendors with patients. Based on the trial results and feedback from nurses and patients, a comprehensive procedure for oral care was developed. This process allowed for the standardization of EBP within the organization, acknowledging the perspectives of the clinical experts, patient preferences, and the research evidence for oral care.

Clinical Nurse Specialist and EBP

A successful strategy used at MGH has been the unit-based clinical nurse specialist. The training of the CNS through the project Retooling for Evidence-Based Nursing Practice has fostered the promotion and the bedside translation of evidence into practice. The MGH EBP is supported and driven by the CNS. At the MGH, CNSs are readily available to nurses to offer expert guidance in patient care. Based on their education and experience, the CNS has advanced skills and knowledge to advance EBP.

The CNSs attend a training program called the Clinical Inquiry Institute. Those who have attended the course praised the program for its content on the fundamentals of EBP and the skill building needed to evaluate evidence to improve patient outcomes. The use of a train-the-trainer model in this project, engaging staff in reflective practice and skills in evaluating the evidence, provided the organization with experts in implementing EBP at the bedside.

Impact of Electronic Medical Record

As MGH integrates an electronic medical record into the organization, this becomes an effective strategy to define the evidence regarding nursing practice. The electronic medical record allows for the use of collected nursing data through the use of standardized nursing language to develop knowledge of the discipline.

The earliest nursing language was the North American Nursing Diagnoses Association (NANDA) nursing diagnoses. Today, there are now 10 distinct vocabularies and 2 different minimum data sets recognized by the American Nurses Association to describe nursing practice (Westra, Delaney, Konicek, & Keenan, 2008). The use of these standardized nursing languages in electronic medical records allows for the delineation of nursing assessment, interventions, and outcomes. The goal in using standardized nursing language is to demonstrate the impact of nursing care on patient outcomes by the analysis of the interoperability of nursing data (Keenan & Wilkie, 2014). The use of standardized nursing language provides the nursing knowledge link to evidence-driven outcomes that accurately reflect the impact that nursing interventions have on patient care. Over time, data from the electronic medical record will link particular patient problems with interventions associated with quality outcomes. This will yield the evidence to build decision support and demonstrate the impact of nursing to high-quality patient care (Jones, Lunney, Keenan, & Moorhead, 2010).

With data from standardized nursing language to describe the patient problems, interventions, and outcomes in the electronic medical record, the next step is the development and testing of decision support systems using these data. These systems will be able to link patient problems to nursing interventions that enhance continuity of care and provide continuously updated data to identify best practices. Nursing care can only be improved when it is described and compared to generate reliable and valid data to develop EBP (Jones et al., 2010). In the recent report *The Future of Nursing: Leading the Change, Advancing Health* (IOM, 2010), the IOM stated that better data collection and improved information infrastructure is required to address the need for evidence to define high-quality, safe, efficient, and effective patient care and to document nursing contribution to patient outcomes.

Summary

An urgent need exists for nursing practice to be evidence based. This requires the commitment of the organization to support an EBP culture through strategies that include clinical evidence, clinical expertise, and knowledge of patient preferences. MGH has implemented multifaceted strategies that acknowledge the need for reflective nursing practice, judicious use of evidence, and knowledge of patient wishes to support a culture of EBP. With the recent call to return to a balance of the tripartite nature of EBP consisting of clinical expertise, evidence, and patient preferences, this organization is using a time-tested model of EBP to support evidence in all its forms to meet the healthcare of our patients (Greenhalgh, Howick, & Maskrey, 2014; Sackett et al., 1996).

References

Agency for Healthcare Research and Quality (AHRQ). (2002). *Systems to rate the strength of scientific evidence-summary.* (The Evidence Report/Technology Assessment No. 47; Publication No. 02-E016). Retrieved from http://archive.ahrq.gov/clinic/epcsums/strength2.htm#Availability

Agency for Healthcare Research and Quality (AHRQ). (2014). National Guideline Clearinghouse. Retrieved from http://www.guideline.gov/

Aiken, L. H., Clarke, S. P., Cheung, R. B., Sloane, D. M., & Silber, J. H. (2003). Educational levels of hospital nurses and surgical patient mortality. *Journal of the American Medical Association, 290,* 1617–1623.

Alston, C., Paget, L., Halsorson, G. C., Novelli, B., Guest, J., McCabe, P., ... Von Kohorn, I. (2012, September). *Communicating with Patients on Health Care Evidence.* Discussion Paper, Institute of Medicine, Washington, DC. Retrieved from http://www.iom.edu/~/media/Files/Perspectives-Files/2012/Discussion-Papers/VSRT-Evidence.pdf

American Association of Critical Care Nurses (AACN). (2011). *AACN Procedure Manual for Critical Care* (6th ed.). St. Louis, MO: Elsevier/Saunders.

American Nurses Association (ANA). (2010a). *Guide to the code of ethics for nurses.* Silver Springs, MD: American Nurses Association.

American Nurses Association (ANA). (2010b). *Nursing: Scope and standards of practice* (2nd ed.). Washington, DC: American Nurses Association.

American Nurses Credentialing Center (ANCC). (2014, August 3). ANCC Magnet Recognition Program®. Retrieved from: http://www.nursecredentialing.org/magnet.aspx

Benner, P. (1984). *From novice to expert: Excellence and power in clinical nursing practice.* Menlo Park, CA: Addison-Wesley.

Benner, P., Tanner, C. A., & Chesla, C. A. (2009). *Expertise in nursing practice: Caring, clinical judgment, and ethics* (2nd ed.). New York, NY: Springer Publishing Company.

Clark, E., Burkett, K., & Stanko-Lopp. (2009). Let evidence guide every new decision (LEGEND): An evidence evaluation system for point-of-care clinicians and guideline development teams. *Journal of Evaluation in Clinical Practice, 15*, 1054–1060.

Coulter, A. (2012). Patient Engagement – what works? *Journal of Ambulatory Care Management 35*(2), 80–89.

Department of Health and Human Services. (2009). *Code of Federal Regulations, Part 46, Protection of Human Subjects.* Retrieved from http://www.hhs.gov/ohrp/humansubjects/guidance/45cfr46.html

Devereaux, P. J., Anderson, D. R., Gardner, M. J., Putnam, W., Flowerdew, G. J., Brownell, B. F., ... Cox, J. L. (2001). Differences between perspectives of physicians and patient on anticoagulation in patients with atrial fibrillation: Observational study. *British Medical Journal, 323*, 1–7.

DiCenso, A., Cullum, N., & Ciliska, D. (1998). Implementing evidence-based nursing: Some misconceptions. *Evidence-Based Nursing 1*, 38–39.

Dykes, P. C., Carroll, D. L., Hurley, A., Lipsitz, S., Benoit, A., Chang, F., ... Middleton, B. (2010). Fall prevention in acute care hospitals: A randomized trial. *Journal of the American Medical Association, 304*, 1912–1918.

Evidence Evaluation Tools & Resources (LEGEND). (2014). Cincinnati Children's, James M. Anderson Center for Health Systems Excellence Retrieved from http://www.cincinnatichildrens.org/service/j/anderson-center/evidence-based-care/legend

Gavigan, A., Cain, C., & Carroll, D. (2014). Effects of informational sessions on anxiety precardiovascular procedure. *Clinical Nursing Research, 23*(3), 281–295.

Green, L., Ottoson, J., Garcia, C., & Hiatt, R. (2009). Diffusion theory and knowledge dissemination, and integration in public health. *Annual Review of Public Health, 30*, 151–174.

Greenhalgh, T., Howick, J., & Maskrey, N. (2014, 27 June). Evidence based medicine: A movement in crisis? *British Medical Journal, 348*: g3725. Retrieved from http://www.bmj.com/content/348/bmj.g3725

Gustafson, D. L. (2005). Transcultural nursing theory from a critical cultural perspective. *Advances in Nursing Science, 28*, 2–16.

Health Resources and Services Administration (HRSA). U.S. Department of Health and Human Service. (2011). *Quality improvement.* Retrieved from http://www.hrsa.gov/quality/toolbox/methodology/qualityimprovement/

Institute of Medicine (IOM). (2000). *To err is human: Building a safer health system.* Washington, DC: National Academies Press.

Institute of Medicine (IOM). (2001). *Crossing the quality chasm: A new health system for the 21st century.* Washington, DC: National Academies Press.

Institute of Medicine (IOM). (2010). *The Future of Nursing: Leading change, advancing health.* Washington, DC: National Academies Press.

James M. Anderson Center for Health Systems Excellence. (2014). Evidence Evaluation Tools & Resources (LEGEND). Retrieved from http://www.cincinnatichildrens.org/service/j/anderson-center/evidence-based-care/legend/

Jenkins, D. A. (1989). Oral care in the ICU: An important nursing role. *Nursing Standard, 4*, 24–29.

Jones, D. A., Lunney, M., Keenan, G., & Moorhead, S. (2010). Standardized nursing language. In A. Debisselle & J. Vessey, *Annual Review of Nursing Research, 28* (pp. 253–293). New York, NY: Springer Publishing.

Kark, V. (2012, 5 July). A lot can be learned from "failed" efforts. Editorial. *Advance for Nurses*. Retrieved from http://Nursing.Advanceweb.Com/Editorial/Content/Printfriendly.Aspx?CC=243302

Keele, R. (2011). *Nursing research and evidence-based practice: Ten steps to success.* Mississauga, Ontario: Jones & Bartlett Learning.

Keenan, G. M., & Wilkie, D. J. (2014). Integration of NNN into EHRS: How are we doing? *International Journal of Nursing Knowledge, 25,* 68–69.

Kutney-Lee, A., Sloane, D. M., & Aiken, L. H. (2013). An increase in the numbers of nurses with a baccalaureate degree is linked to lower rates of postsurgery mortality. *Health Affairs, 32,* 579–586.

Lee, S. M., & Brandt, L. (2013). Evidence/knowledge driven practice. In J. I. Erickson, D. A. Jones, & M. Ditomassi (Eds.), *Fostering Nurse-Led Care: Professional Practice for the Bedside Leader from Massachusetts General Hospital* (pp. 217–239). Indianapolis, IN: Sigma Theta Tau International.

Lenburg, C. B. (2011). The influence of contemporary trends and issues on nursing education. In B. Cherry & S. R. Jacob (Eds.), *Contemporary Nursing: Issues, Trends, & Management* (5th ed.) (pp.41–70). St. Louis, MO: Mosby.

Luzinski, C. (2011). The Magnet® Model: An infrastructure for excellence. *Journal of Nursing Administration, 41,* 441–442.

MacLean, S., Mulla, S., Akl, E. A., Jankowski, M., Vandvik, P. O., Ebrahim, ... Guyatt, G. H. (2012). Patient values and preferences in decision making for antithrombotic therapy: A systematic review. *CHEST, 141*(2 Supplement), e1S-23S. Retrieved from http://journal.publications.chestnet.org/data/Journals/CHEST/23443/112290.pdf

Marra, A. R., Cal, R. G., Silva, C. V, Caserta, R. A., Paes, D. T., Maura, D. F, Jr., ... Durao, M. S.(2009). Successful prevention of ventilator-associated pneumonia in an intensive care setting. *American Journal of Infection Control, 37,* 619–625.

McClosky, D. J. (2008). Nurses' perceptions of research utilization in a corporate health care system. *Journal of Nursing Scholarship, 40,* 39–45.

McHugh, M. D., & Lake, E. T. (2010). Understanding clinical expertise: Nurse education, experience, and the hospital context. *Research in Nursing & Health, 33,* 276–287.

Melnyk, B. M., Fineout-Overholt, E., Stillwell. S. B., & Williamson, K. M. (2009). Igniting a spirit of inquiry: An essential foundation for evidence-based practice. *American Journal of Nursing, 109*(11), 49–52.

Morse, J. M. (2008). *Preventing patient falls: Establishing a fall intervention program* (2nd ed.). New York, NY: Springer.

Munro, C., Grap, M. J., Jones, D. J., McClish, D. K., & Sessler, C. N. (2009). Chlorhexidine, tooth brushing, and preventing ventilator-associated pneumonia in critically ill adults. *American Journal of Critical Care, 18,* 428–437.

Nelsey, L. (1986). Mouth care and the intubated patient: The aim of preventing infection. *Intensive Care Nursing, 1,* 187–193.

Newhouse, R. P. (2007). Creating the infrastructure supportive of evidence-based nursing practice: Leadership strategies. *Worldviews of Evidence-Based Practice, 4,* 21–29.

Newhouse, R. P., & Pettit, J. C. (2006). The slippery slope: Differentiating between quality improvement and research. *Journal of Nursing Administration, 36*, 211–219.

Nowak, T. T., (2005). Vietnamese. In J. Lipson & S. Dibble (Eds.), *Culture & Clinical Care* (pp. 446–460). San Francisco, CA: UCSF Nursing Press.

Oxman, A. D., Sackett, D. L., & Guyatt, G. H. (1993). Users' guides to the medical literature: I. How to get started. *Journal of the American Medical Association, 207*, 2093–2095.

Porter-O'Grady, T. (2001). Is shared governance still relevant? *Journal of Nursing Administration, 31*, 468–473.

Restrepo, P., Jameson, D. L., & Carroll, D. L. (2015). Improving deep vein thrombosis prophylaxis with mechanical modalities in surgical intensive care unit. *Journal of Nursing Care Quality, 30*, 31-37.

Sackett, D. L., Rosenberg, W. M. C., Muir Gray, J. A., Harnes, R. B., & Richardson, W. S. (1996). Evidence based medicine: What it is and what it isn't. *British Medical Journal, 312*, 71–72.

Stanley, T., Sitterding, M., Broome, M. E., & McCaskey, M. (2011). Engaging and developing research leaders in practice: Creating a foundation for a culture of clinical inquiry. *Journal of Pediatric Nursing, 26*, 480–488.

Titler, M. G. (2008). The evidence for evidence-based practice implementation. In R. Hughes (Ed.), *Patient safety and quality: An evidence-based handbook for nurses.* (AHRQ Publication No. 08 0043). Rockville, MD: Agency for Healthcare Research and Quality. Retrieved from http://www.ncbi.nlm.nih.gov/books/NBK2659/

Titler, M. G., Kleiber, C., Steelman, V. J. Rakel, B. A., Budreau, G., Everett, L. Q., ... Goode, C. J. (2001). The Iowa model of evidence-based practice to promote quality care. *Critical Care Nursing Clinics of North America, 13*, 497–509.

Watson, F., & Rebair, A. (2014). The art of noticing: essential to nursing practice. *British Journal of Nursing, 23*, 514–517.

Webb, J. J. (2011). Nursing research and evidence-based practice. In B. Cherry & S. R. Jacob (Eds.), *Contemporary Nursing: Issues, Trends, & Management* (5th ed.) (pp. 101–121). St. Louis, MO: Mosby.

Westra, B. L., Delaney, C. W., Konicek, D., & Keenan, G. (2008). Nursing standards to support the electronic health record. *Nursing Outlook, 56*, 258–266.

Wolf, G., Triolo, P., & Ponte, P. R. (2008). Magnet Recognition Program®: The next generation. *Journal of Nursing Administration, 38*, 200–204.

Chapter 5

Supporting Operational Effectiveness and Encouraging Research Through Innovation

–Jeffrey M. Adams, PhD, RN
–Jeanette Ives Erickson, DNP, RN, NEA-BC, FAAN
–Marianne Ditomassi, DNP, MBA, RN
–Dorothy A. Jones, EdD, RN, FAAN, FNI

Healthcare leaders are searching for ways to create new synergies and efficiencies in today's complex health environments to enhance patient care, education, and research and to nurture collaborative and rewarding professional practice environments (Ives Erickson, Ditomassi, & Jones, 2008). At Massachusetts General Hospital (MGH), innovation is an integral component of the Professional Practice Model (PPM) (Chapter 8, "Evaluating Professional Practice in Nursing Research"). The MGH PPM serves as the framework to align clinicians and others as we seek to enhance care that ensures patient care delivery and associated structures meet the healthcare needs of the patients served.

This chapter examines the creation of a vision and subsequent strategies to promote innovation and discovery for the purposes of redesigning care that is safe, of the highest quality, efficient, and equitable. Moreover, the goal is that the care be delivered in a timely, efficient, and effective manner that is relationship based with patients, families, and within the care team.

The term *innovation* has a variety of definitions. Blakeney, Carleton, McCarthy, and Coakley (2009) define innovation as a process for inventing something new or improving on that which already exists. Greenhalgh (2004, p. 581) describes innovation as follows:

> *"A novel set of behaviors, routines, and ways of working that are directed at improving health outcomes, administrative efficiency, cost effectiveness, or users' experience and that are implemented by planned and coordinated actions."*

The American Nurses Credentialing Center adopted this as the guiding definition for the conduct, review, and evaluation of innovation in Magnet®-recognized hospitals.

At MGH, we embrace this definition. Our goals for innovation include the development, implementation, and evaluation of discipline-specific and interdisciplinary interventions, changes in care delivery, and application of evidence-based practice.

Innovation at MGH

Established in 2006, the Center for Innovation in Care Delivery (Center for Innovation), at MGH, was built to foster innovative interdisciplinary practice (Ives Erickson, Ditomassi, & Jones, 2008). The vision evolved as we searched for new ways to address the challenges in healthcare, with an emphasis on enhancing cost-effective care. Today, the Center for Innovation is a center within the Institute for Patient Care (see Chapter 2, "Creating an Infrastructure that Enhances Professional Practice"), which emphasizes this forward-thinking vision that supports transdisciplinary efforts toward the development, advancement, and interrelated nature of innovative products and processes. Guided by both abstract and practical components, the Center for Innovation provides a *think and do tank* for uniting organizational efforts designed for rapid cycle change that advances care redesign efforts on behalf of our patients and their families.

The goal of the Center for Innovation is to provide the support and resources needed to encourage and develop innovation in clinical practice. Its leaders articulate the center's instrumental role in helping clinicians from multiple disciplines access the resources and partnerships they need to explore ideas for innovation and to translate those into practice. Through the center, interdisciplinary resources in education and research can be optimally matched with opportunities to impact patient care. The Center for Innovation provides a more efficient way for us to chronicle, study, and advance the innovations that occur at the bedside in all areas of clinical practice.

The center's aim is to introduce into the environment new and creative processes/products that result in changes and improve outcomes. For healthcare, innovation is an encompassing idea that allows for the realization of visionary leaders and staff to introduce into an already complex environment changes that will alter the way things are *usually* done. The design and implementation strategies needed to implement change require as much thought and planning as the innovation itself. Careful testing and evaluation is critical to the process.

It was important to us to graphically define the center as we communicated the opportunities to clinical staff. Our goal was to have clinicians identify clinical problems that needed to be addressed in new ways, especially when other efforts had failed. We wanted to design an approach that allowed everyone a unique opportunity to step forward with ideas that would challenge the status quo and create new opportunities for growth. Figure 5.1 is a representative model of the work and philosophy of the Center for Innovation.

At the far left in Figure 5.1, you can see a list of disciplinary domains of practice comprising Patient Care Services at MGH, from Nursing to Speech-Language Pathology. At the right of the figure, you can see each individual discipline's approach to innovation, with a unique discipline-specific perspective represented through an overarching and unifying lens of the organization. The importance of having a consilient vision, or linking together multiple disciplines' perspectives, is further understood within the framework of a professional practice model, which influences a positive professional practice environment essential to continuously fostering the existence and betterment of the other, as represented in the oval in Figure 5.1.

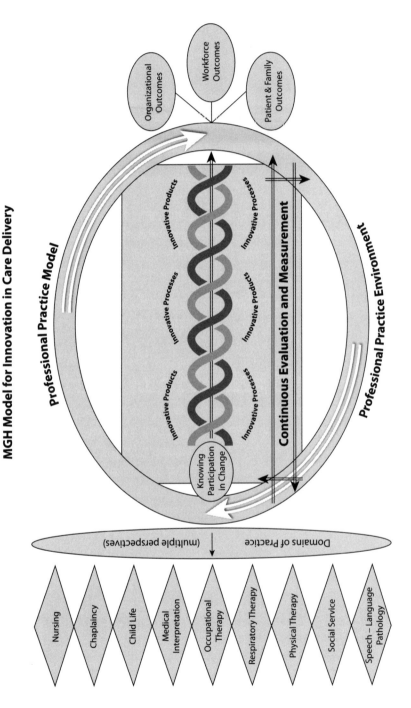

FIGURE 5.1

MGH Model for Innovation in Care Delivery

Entering the oval at the far left of Figure 5.1, innovation is promoted within a learning environment guided by the belief that when knowledge is available to all clinicians they become active participants in decisions about change and engage more freely and knowingly in the change process (Barrett, 2003). The partnership between the provider and the change or innovation that occurs helps to motivate staff to sustain changes and become part of the ongoing development of innovative products and processes. Within Figure 5.1, the interrelationship of innovation products and processes is represented as a braid. This innovation braid reflects the continuous overlap of the generation of innovative products and the identification of innovative processes whereby improvements in one aspect of innovation can create the stimulus or opportunity to improve the other.

The continuous and dynamic evaluation of the innovation experience is represented as a rectangle and includes understanding the dimensions within the professional practice model, the professional practice environment, innovative products, and innovative processes. This approach is essential to effectively measure impact, sustain change, and optimize outcomes within the organization, the workforce, and patients and families (depicted at the far right of Figure 5.1). This model helped to clarify the mission of the Center for Innovation and guide how our staff could participate in or design new discoveries.

Development of Innovative Products

The Center for Innovation actively works with clinical staff involved in multiple organizational roles and who possess a variety of skill sets, knowledge, and experiences. In addition, the center has established partnerships with outside organizations, universities, and communities to promote the development of innovative product, for example design, patenting, licensing. Through collaboration with area experts existent within the MGH system, innovation becomes an important catalyst for change. The center's leader works with the MGH workforce, our patients, and several collaborative groups. These collaborations have resulted in the generation of myriad ideas:

- Staff development of innovative product ideas currently in nondisclosure status. These product ideas span various areas, including physical therapy, phlebotomy, and urologic nursing being developed/explored as potential revenue-generation streams.

- Advisement to local middle school students on an award-winning Google Glass application for their visually impaired classmate to access "a set of eyes" via a cell phone application (Annear, 2014). This advisement realized two goals: community goodwill and investment in the next generation of scientists.

- The Massachusetts Institute of Technology (MIT) for Soldier Nanotechnologies on translational applications of future battlefield care; current to near-future care delivery innovation products for remote monitoring and medication delivery (Adams et al., 2011) as part of keeping an eye toward the future of care delivery.

The challenge of developing products within the operational setting of patient care becomes a delicate balance of keeping an eye on "innovations as the next great thing" (Adams, 2014) and adequate and judicious application of resources to address needs in the near future. It is necessary not only to sustain and justify results but also to envision and guide the far-future models of the care delivery environment. While there is much excitement and value around the development of innovative products, as leaders focus on identifying the next great processes or model of care delivery, the development of innovative initiatives that address the *current* needs in healthcare is equally important.

Creation of Innovative Processes

As has been well documented in the literature (Social Security Advisory Board, 2009), models of care that have existed for more than a century are no longer sustainable in today's rapidly changing healthcare environment. In efforts to address this needed change, work was undertaken at the Institute for Healthcare

Improvement under then CEO and Founder Donald Berwick, MD, MPP, (2008). What emerged was the Triple Aim. The tenants of the Triple Aim include:

- Increase care quality

- Increase access to populations

- Decrease cost

In 2010, following Berwick's appointment by President Barack Obama to serve as the administrator of the Centers for Medicare & Medicaid Services (CMS), the Triple Aim concepts became a cornerstone of the CMS vision (CMS, 2012; Fleming, 2010), and the CMS Innovation Solution Center was established.

CMS Advisors Program

Our formative years launching the Innovation Center led us to be one of 75 organizations invited to participate in the CMS Advisors Program (CMS, 2014). The CMS Advisors Program was designed to create partnerships to identify and test new models of care delivery in their own organizations and create partnerships to find new ideas that work and share them regionally and across the United States. In this capacity, and guided by the goals of the Triple Aim, MGH spearheaded an innovative project titled "Door to Chemo Hang Time" to address an identified opportunity stemming from three delays in care for the population receiving chemotherapy:

- Blood work and chemotherapy orders were not always completed upon admission.

- Pharmacy preparation, including hydration, pre-medications, and chemotherapy, was not completed as a single order

- Long waits occurred for insertion of a peripherally inserted central catheter (PICC line) at the time of admission.

The project was designed to improve patient experience, decrease cost, and increase access, capacity, and throughput via consolidation and expedition of known processes, and thus the "Door to Chemo Hang Time" addressed each of the Triple Aim concepts.

American Organization of Nurse Executives – Care Innovation and Transformation

Additionally, MGH participated in the American Organization of Nurse Executives – Care Innovation and Transformation (AONE-CIT) (Caramanica & Stefancyk, 2012, p. 22) project on a women's health oncology unit. The AONE-CIT program is designed to facilitate ownership of practice at the bedside by providing staff with tangible tools and teaching them via real-time application how to impact practice at the bedside. AONE-CIT at MGH was embraced, and more than 20 small tests of change were implemented by staff. Projects ranged from implementation of in-room pill cutters, to teatime with the chaplains, to quiet-at-night initiatives. Outcomes of this work are being prepared for publication, which will chronicle the experiences, changes, and outcomes proved to be of benefit to patients, staff, and leadership participating in these efforts.

Transforming Care at the Bedside

MGH also participated in the Transforming Care at the Bedside (TCAB) initiative, which was a precursor to the AONE-CIT program. TCAB was a national program designed by the Institute for Healthcare Improvement (IHI) and disseminated by the Robert Wood Johnson Foundation and the American Organization of Nurse Executives (AONE) to provide nurses at the bedside with tools to improve efficiency. The program taught a specific methodology for process improvement. MGH joined the third round of TCAB hospitals. During the 2-year study (2007–2009), clinical nurses on a General Medicine unit conducted 33 tests of change and adopted 11 of those (Stefancyk, 2008).

The TCAB project created sustainable practices on the General Medicine unit. One pertained to an MGH tradition called *green books*, three-ring binders where much of the relevant clinical information is kept. Nurses reported a "morning rush" to access the green books (vital signs from the previous shift and so forth) by several groups of clinicians: interns, nurses, student nurses, and patient care associates (PCAs), all needing the same information at the same time and from the same source.

To create a win-win, the TCAB clinical nurses devised a new plan that decreased the competition for the information. After some consideration, the nurses proposed that they, not the interns, would present the patient's case information at morning rounds. This would free up the interns from needing to access the green books. This simple change created a culture change in several ways:

- The clinical nurses accessed what they needed and then gave the green books to the PCAs, who could then begin their early morning activities (specifically, vital signs).

- It placed the clinical nurses into morning rounds, where they would not only provide patients' information but could also influence the plan of care for the day. Rounds developed into a venue of greater knowledge sharing, clinical nurses better understood the plan of care, and PCAs got the information they needed.

The CNO, highly enthusiastic about TCAB, stated:

> "TCAB embraces a new way of thinking about care delivery. The goal is to empower nurses and other frontline staff to have a voice in unit-based systems—to tap into the knowledge and experience of direct caregivers and use that knowledge to re-design care-delivery models. In that respect, according to the Institute for Healthcare Improvement, TCAB 'does not simply fine-tune the status quo, but rather transforms the elements that affect care, including: care-delivery processes, nursing care models, the physical environment, organizational culture and norms, collaboration, and performance.' In short, TCAB encourages nurses and other team members to quickly identify, test, and then implement new ideas based on their perceptions and observations at the bedside. And who better to make those important decisions than direct-care providers?"(Ives Erickson, 2012, p. 436)

The Process of Evaluating Innovation

Identification of essential data to be collected, stored, and retrieved over time is critical to realizing the sustainability and impact of initiatives. When multiple groups (disciplines, patients, and families) as well as the organizational infrastructure are engaged in innovation implementation, preparation of the people involved, support, coaching, and resources are critical to the success of the effort. The development of an evaluation plan early in the process can facilitate data collection and begin to map out the questions, evaluation design, and data needed to monitor the effectiveness and overall impact of innovation immediately and over time.

Implementing innovative ideas and evaluating the impact within the care delivery setting is optimal when a wide range of measures and data is collected longitudianally (with consistent repetitive inquiry) and near real-time dissemination of results to all relevant groups. Data resulting from innovation evaluation within a care delivery setting are often not conclusive in themselves. Findings must be evaluated at selected times following the introduction of the innovation and explored both clinically and statistically to determine significance and overall data trending. However, because of the need for frequent and repetitive inquiry and reporting of data, innovation evaluation over short time periods does identify trends and offer directional support to inform knowledge-based operational decisions and ask new questions to expand future data analysis (Adams, 2014).

Formalizing an innovation process evaluation plan in a care delivery setting is in itself a learning process that can occur over several years. It requires both long-term and short-term planning. In addition, it involves a commitment to establishing needed resources to coordinate adequate data collection, storage, retrieval mechanisms, and governance. It also involves recognition that all initiatives, big and small, need to be evaluated with pre- and post-measures so that the data is available for large-scale organizational evaluation efforts that address for example impact, sustainability, and relationship between and among variables being evaluated. For organizations on such a journey, it is the inclusion of strategic planning efforts and access to needed resources that truly optimizes the influence of innovation across populations and organizational settings.

The commitment to engage in innovation evaluation requires a focus on the system's ability to do the following:

- Collect, store, and retrieve data

- Provide statistical support for design analysis

- Coordinate efforts to make meaning of the results

- Disseminate, under a specific strategy, knowledge generated from the findings to guide change and promote learning of benefit to others

As an organization approaches innovation evaluation, many factors are essential, including the selection of the intervention or multiple innovations, the timing of implementation, the determination of pre-testing measures, as well as data management and storage and statistical support.

Innovation Unit Initiative Evaluation

An example of our innovation evaluation work was a project called "The Evaluation of the MGH Innovation Unit Initiative (IU)." Launched in 2012, MGH IUs were intended to be testing grounds for change—a strategic initiative designed to create an environment for the timely trial of new ideas. The initiative began with 12 inpatient units, and in 2013, more inpatient units were added as part of Phases II and III of the rollout. As of this writing, 41 inpatient units are designated as IUs. With the collaboration of the Munn Center, an evaluation plan was developed and implemented.

The Patient's Journey

In the inpatient setting, IUs centered on the patient's journey. Figure 5.2 depicts the process of care before, during, and after hospitalization.

At the heart of the IU initiative are 15 interventions that were generated by staff and leadership throughout Nursing and Patient Care Services and the hospital at large (see Table 5.1). These interventions represent top-priority actions aimed at achieving the highest level of consistency, continuity, and efficiency. Continuity is enhanced by standardization wherever possible.

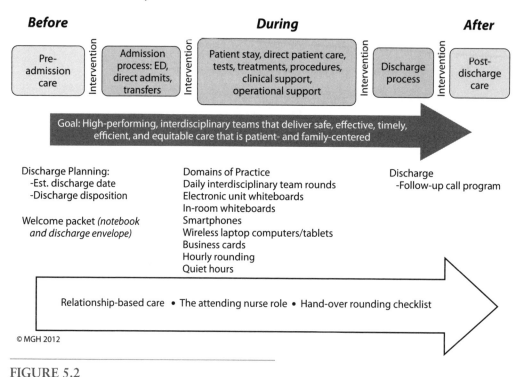

Innovations in Care Delivery
"Patient Journey" Framework: Initial 15 Interventions

FIGURE 5.2

Innovation Journey

TABLE 5.1   Innovation Bundle Phase 1 Interventions and Definitions

INNOVATION UNITS	15 INTERVENTIONS
Relationship-Based Care	Support and strengthen the relationships with ourselves, patient, and team; this is the basis for the care we provide (Manthey, 2006).
Attending Nurse Role	Oversee the continuity and progression of the overall patient/family plan of care from admission to discharge (Ives Erickson, Ditomassi, & Adams, 2012).

INNOVATION UNITS	15 INTERVENTIONS
Handover Communication	Improve quality of care, efficiency, and outcomes using a structured, reliable handover process during care transitions (Adams & Osborne-McKenzie, 2012).
Estimated Discharge Date	Articulate estimated discharge date and disposition upon admission.
Welcome Packet	Create welcome packet (that includes patient/ family notebook and discharge envelope) to support communication.
Domains of Practice	Ensure across-the-board understanding of each discipline's domain of practice (Fairman, Rowe, Hassmiller, & Shalala, 2011).
Interdisciplinary Team Rounds	Implement daily interdisciplinary team rounds to coordinate patient care (O'Leary, Sehgal, Terrell, & Williams, 2012).
Electronic Whiteboards	Install electronic unit whiteboards.
In-Room Patient Whiteboards	Install in-room whiteboards to enhance communication among caregiver team, patient, and family.
Smartphone Technology	Introduce smartphone technology for unit staff (Voalté) that expedites communication among the team.
Wireless Laptops	Provide staff with access to portable wireless tablets or computers.
ARN Business Cards	Equip attending nurses with business cards to ensure optimal communication and continuity.
Hourly Rounding	Implement hourly rounding with the four P's: presence, pain, positioning, and personal hygiene (Rondinelli, Ecker, Crawford, Seelinger, & Omery, 2012).

continues

TABLE 5.1 *continued*

INNOVATION UNITS	15 INTERVENTIONS
Quiet Hours	Implement quiet hours to promote rest and healing (Boehm & Morast, 2009).
Discharge Phone Calls	Implement discharge follow-up phone calls to clarify questions about discharge plan (Cochran, Blair, Wissinger, & Nuss, 2012).

Evaluation Framework

Like the innovation unit program itself, the approach to the evaluation of innovation was multifaceted and produced great opportunity for learning, refinement, and growth. Because the implementation of the innovation program occurred in several phases, with growth and adjustment at each phase, the evaluation planning and strategy were also regularly reviewed and refined to further meet the needs of the organization. The initial 15 interventions as listed in Table 5.1 were implemented on Phase 1 units and evaluated as part of the innovation evaluation program; they are represented in the second box from the left in Figure 5.3, where the evaluation data sources are noted in the box on the far right of Figure 5.3.

Innovation Unit Evaluation Design

The evaluation of this complex innovation program centered on the following research questions:

- Are IUs effective in improving outcomes for patients, staff, and the organization?

- What is the general experience of working on / receiving care on an IU?

- Does the role of the attending registered nurse (ARN) impact care and how so?

Innovation Unit Schema

Innovation Cluster Focus Areas*	Interventions**	Evaluation (Pre, During, Post)	
		Quantitative	Qualitative
Quality of Care	_Throughout Admission_	• HCAHPS	• Focus Groups (Staff, Patients, Families, etc.)
	Relationship-Based Care	• Leadership Influence Over Professional Practice Environments (LIPPES)	• Observations
Patient Experience	Attending Nurse Handover Rounding Checklist		• Survey of the Innovation Unit Expectations (SIUE-pre)
	Pre-Admission	• LOS	
	Pre-Admit Data Collection Welcome Packet	• Quality Indicators	• Survey of the Innovation Unit Experiences (SIUE-post)
Workforce Satisfaction	_During Admission_	• Patients' Perceptions of Feeling Known (PPFKN)	
	Domains of Practice Interdisciplinary Rounds Business Cards Quiet Hours Hourly Rounding Electronic White Boards In-Room White Boards Smart Phones Handheld Tablets	• Readmissions	
Cost		• Revised Perceptions of Practice Environment Scale (RPPE)	
	Post-Discharge Discharge Follow-up Phone Calls	• Cost per Case Mix	
*The clusters are a lens with which we gain perspective on any particular intervention.	_Others as identified_	• Staff Retention	
		Other measures as identified	

© Massachusetts General Hospital 2015   **May apply to any or all 3 of the cluster focus areas   February 2015

FIGURE 5.3
Phase 1 Innovation Evaluation Plan

- Is there a relationship between and among interventions and outcomes?

- What are the staff perceptions of each intervention on cost, quality and safety, and patient and staff satisfaction?

- Are the interventions sustained over time?

Data Collection

In addressing these questions, the evaluation team purposefully expanded the breadth of evaluation approach, acknowledging that if a significant finding was identified in any of the results, a deeper dive into the data was then available and warranted. It has been expressed as broad with the ability to address specificity as needed. In this vein, we captured multiple and consistent measures, including the following:

- Administrative data such as HCAHPS (Hospital Consumer Assessment of Healthcare Providers and Systems) patient satisfaction data, length of stay, and cost measures and quality indicators collected as part of regular operations

- Focus group data designed to understand the experiences of implementing the innovation unit program

- Staff surveys developed to capture expectations, experiences, and perceptions of the professional practice environment in which staff work, and leaders' perceptions of their ability to influence the environment they oversee

- Patient surveys aimed at understanding their perceptions of feeling known by their nurses, mailers, observations, and analysis of quality and administrative data (Adams & Jones, 2012)

Data collection methods were intended to cast a wide net and allow for multiple inquiries as research questions were identified.

Data Analysis

Our data collection and analysis approach led to some important findings specific to each intervention, including the following:

- The new role of the ARN was universally viewed as a positive change.

- ARNs self-identified as having an increased job satisfaction.

Focus group findings suggested:

- Communication seen as improving across and within disciplines and telephone follow-up calls were met with a positive response from patients and clinicians.

- Interdisciplinary rounding was viewed as a positive to enhance "knowing" the patient.

- The in-room whiteboards were celebrated as especially effective when identifying patient goals and discharge dates. The data confirmed that strong unit leadership positively affected outcomes at the unit level.

- New wireless phones (Voalté) were identified as a universal success because they enhance nurse communication. They also decreased overhead paging and, coupled with the quiet-hours intervention, were repeatedly acknowledged as effective in optimizing the quiet-at-night component of the patient experience.

Some challenges were also identified that helped reframe and improve the innovation unit program:

- Initially, ARNs were given laptops to enhance mobile documentation; however, they were widely identified as heavy and not necessary for the ARN role. Therefore, they were eliminated.

- There was an expressed difficulty maintaining the original model of a 5 days a week/8 hour a day schedule for ARNs. Each focus group spoke of the pace of change, suggesting that that the accelerated rate of change was challenging.

- Electronic whiteboards were designed and conceptualized for use as patient bed locators, but this intervention proved to be delayed, conflicting with a new electronic health record (EHR) implementation.

As the team continued to refine and optimize resources and efforts surrounding innovation, gaps in the continuum of care and the expertise of all clinical disciplines to improve the patient experience, quality of care, and staff satisfaction and empowerment, while decreasing redundancy, costs, length of stay, and readmission rates (Ives Erickson et al., 2012) were evaluated. The initial evaluation focused on the collection of a broad range of data using multiple methods (e.g., qualitative, descriptive, and quantitative) to tell the innovation story.

During the early part of the program's data collection and analysis, the differences between research and evaluation became increasingly clear. Specifically, as part of operations in a care delivery setting, innovation evaluation is enhanced by broad, frequent, repetitive inquiry and near real-time dissemination of findings. The need to streamline and produce the knowledge of "how we're doing rebuilding the ship, while the ship is sailing" became increasingly apparent.

The innovative process evaluation is, in and of itself, unique, in that it provides insight for actionable decision-making that often leads to research based on longitudinal findings. More specifically, our refined approach includes a 90-day innovation cycle, as follows:

- A 30-day implementation window

- A 30-day rumination/settling-in window

- A 30-day evaluation/reporting window

This 90-day cycle stems from work by Proctor and Gamble (Huston & Sakkab, 2006), and was later used in healthcare at the IHI (2012) as part of those organizations' innovations work. The 90-day cycle can be repeated, thus supporting quarterly reporting to assist in identifying trends promptly and accelerating or course correcting as needed (Adams, 2014).

Evaluating the Relationships Between Evaluation Components

Following the launch of Phase 1 innovation units and the implementation of interventions intended to continually improve patient satisfaction, quality of care, and cost, a detailed evaluation ensued. While in the adult inpatient setting, each of the components of the patient experience, also known as HCAHPS, showed a clinically significant positive trend post-intervention (Ives Erickson, 2014, pp. 2–3), and the overall rating showed a statistically significant increase following the implementation of the innovation unit interventions.

Additionally interesting and important, the presence of professional practice environment components, such as clinician control over practice, conflict management, teamwork, and better RN-MD relationships, may actually accelerate innovation. Similarly, leadership seemingly matters in making innovation happen. When unit leaders expressed having a more collegial administrative approach, greater internal strategy and resolve, high expectations of staff, and increased authority innovation was accelerated.

In addition, innovation quality efforts, such as improving (or eliminating) central line infections, pressure ulcers, and/or fall rates, happen faster in the presence of:

- Components of an increasingly positive professional practice environment

- Components of leadership perceptions, with increased influence over the practice environment that they oversee

The team is continuously evaluating the successes, challenges, adoption, and sustainability of innovative initiatives, telling the story in context of the immediate, while tracking longitudinally for opportunity for specified research. In the era of big data, and these longitudinal innovation projects, we have increasingly learned the importance of collecting, merging, managing, cleaning, analyzing, and sustaining a longitudinal data set. Moving forward we face various challenges related to the coordination of the data from various sources, including server space for storage of the data and synchronizing when updates/corrections/clarifications are made to the data sets (something that happens regularly in hospitals).

Summary

Evaluating the processes of innovation within a care delivery setting is and has been a learning experience for all involved. As documented within this chapter, innovation evaluation at MGH has been a stepwise process, providing a resource for others seeking to innovate. Innovation evaluation is as much about learning, adapting, and, when necessary, abandoning as it is about finding the successes as you build toward organizational excellence.

References

Adams, J. M. (2014). Guest Editorial: How do we know if we're innovating? A strategy for innovation evaluation in a practice setting. *Journal of Nursing Administration, 44*(2), 63-64.

Adams, J. M., Failano, R., Bordetsky, A. R., Elman, N., Bourakov, E., & Aspell Adams, A. (2011). Setting the stage for the future of care delivery: Civilian implications for emerging battlefield care technologies. *AONE Voice,* November.

Adams, J.M., & Jones, D.A. (2012). Evaluating change on innovation units. *Caring Headlines,* November 1, 15.

Adams, J. M., & Osborne-McKenzie, T. (2012). Advancing the evidence base for standardized provider handover structure: Using staff nurse descriptions for information needed to deliver competent care. *Journal of Continuing Education in Nursing, 43*(6), 261-266.

Annear, D. (2014). Meet the new class of high tech innovation. Retrieved from http://www.bostonmagazine.com/news/blog/2014/02/07/mccall-middle-school-app-challenge/

Barrett, E. A. M. (2003). Update on a measure of power as knowing participation in change. In O. L. Strickland & C. DiIorio (Eds.), *Measurement of nursing outcomes: Focus on patient/client outcomes (Vol. 4).* New York: Springer, 21-39.

Berwick, D. (2008). Triple Aim: Care, health, and cost. *Health Affairs, 27*(3), 759-769.

Blakeney, B., Carleton, P., McCarthy, C., & Coakley, E. (2009). Unlocking the power of innovation. *The Online Journal of Issues in Nursing, 14*(2).

Boehm, H., & Morast, S. (2009). Quiet time. *American Journal of Nursing, 109*(11), 49-52.

Caramanica, L., & Stefancyk, A. (2012). Focus on AONE Center for Care Innovation and Transformation. *AONE Voice,* September 1.

Centers for Medicare & Medicaid Services (CMS). (2012). Our innovation models. Retrieved from http://innovation.cms.gov/

Centers for Medicare & Medicaid Services (CMS). (2014). Innovation advisor. Retrieved from http://innovation.cms.gov/initiatives/Innovation-Advisors-Program/#collapse-tableDetails

Cochran, V. Y., Blair, B., Wissinger, L., & Nuss, T. D. (2012). Lessons learned from implementation of postdischarge telephone calls at Baylor Health Care System. *Journal of Nursing Administration, 42*(1), 40-46.

Fairman, J. A., Rowe, J. W., Hassmiller, S., & Shalala, D. E. (2011). Broadening the scope of nursing practice. *The New England Journal of Medicine, 364*(3), 193-196.

Fleming, C. (2010). Berwick brings the 'Triple Aim' to CMS. Retrieved from http://healthaffairs.org/blog/2010/09/14/berwick-brings-the-triple-aim-to-cms/

Greenhalgh, T. (2004). Diffusion of innovations in service organizations: Systematic review and recommendations. *The Milbank Quarterly, 82,* 581-629.

Huston, L, & Sakkab, N. (2006). Connect and develop. *Harvard Business Review*, March, 58-66.

Institute for Healthcare Improvement (IHI). (2012). 90-Day Innovation Process. Retrieved from http://www.ihi.org/about/Documents/IHI%20Innovation%20Summary.pdf

Ives Erickson, J. (2012). MGH Magnet® evidence, NK 8, Submitted to the American Nurses Credentialing Center.

Ives Erickson, J. (2014). Now more than ever: Innovation units are key: Helping to make care more effective, efficient, and affordable. *Caring Headlines,* October, 2-3.

Ives Erickson, J., Ditomassi, M., & Adams, J. M. (2012). Innovations in care delivery: A blueprint for the future. *Nursing Economic$, 30*(5), 282-287.

Ives Erickson, J., Ditomassi, M, & Jones, D. (2008). Interdisciplinary institute for patient care: advancing clinical excellence. *Journal of Nursing Administration, 38*(6), 308-314.

Ives Erickson, J, Ditomassi, M., & Jones, D. (2013). *Fostering nurse-led care at the bedside: Professional practice for the bedside leader from Massachusetts General Hospital.* Indianapolis, IN: Sigma Theta Tau International.

Manthey, M. (2006). Leadership for relationship-based care. *Creative Nursing, 12*(1), 10-11.

O'Leary, K. J., Sehgal, N. L., Terrell, G., & Williams, M. V. (2012). Interdisciplinary teamwork in hospitals: A review and practical recommendations or improvement, *Journal of Hospital Medicine, 7*(1), 48-54.

Rondinelli, J., Ecker, M., Crawford, C., Seelinger, C., & Omery, A. (2012). Hourly rounding implementation. *Journal of Nursing Administration, 42*(6), 326-332.

Social Security Advisory Board (SSAB). (2009). The unsustainable cost of health care. Retrieved from http://www.ssab.gov/documents/TheUnsustainableCostofHealthCare_508.pdf

Stefancyk, A. L. (2008). Transforming care at Mass General. *American Journal of Nursing, 108*(9), 71-72.

Chapter 6

Promoting Nursing Research in a Multidisciplinary Organization

–Sara E. Dolan Looby, PhD, ANP-BC, FAAN

Nursing research is an integral component of the research infrastructure in multidisciplinary organizations. The continually increasing number of nurses with research-intensive doctoral preparation working in clinical practice, along with the growth of nursing science and increased expertise in use of existing and creative methodologies to study phenomena of concern to the discipline, has resulted in a growing visibility of nurse scientists/researchers in the practice environment and increases in funding opportunities from governmental and other sources.

As the impact of nursing research and evidence-driven care continues to influence patient care and related outcomes, the opportunities to participate in collaborative initiatives with other disciplines will grow. The introduction of creative research strategies that offer perspectives from a variety of disciplines is needed to advance patient care and manage the economic challenges faced by multidisciplinary organizations in this ever-changing healthcare environment. Nurse scientists have expertise in a variety of research methods, including qualitative and quantitative research, and in diverse programs of research designed to enhance patient-centered care, safety, and quality of life throughout the lifespan.

This chapter provides an overview of the research infrastructure at Massachusetts General Hospital (MGH) and nursing's presence within this infrastructure. Interdisciplinary opportunities to enhance research development and strategies for increasing visibility of nursing research within a multidisciplinary organization are also presented.

Nursing Presence Within the Research Infrastructure

MGH has the largest hospital-based research program in the United States ("Facts at a Glance," n.d.) and is the leading National Institutes of Health (NIH) funding recipient among independent hospitals ("Overview and History," n.d.). Research Management and the Executive Committee on Research (ECOR) lead the research enterprise at MGH (see Table 6.1). Research Management serves as the executive branch and oversees research policy and operations, and ECOR is the legislative branch that provides guidance on research growth, education, development, and policies (ECOR). ECOR has both voting and nonvoting members from the MGH community who serve on subcommittees to help oversee and implement its policies and initiatives.

TABLE 6.1   MGH Research Infrastructure and Collaborators

NAME	WEBSITE
MGH Research & Research Management	http://www.massgeneral.org/research/about/
Executive Committee on Research	http://ecor.mgh.harvard.edu/
Partners Human Research Committee	https://partnershealthcare-public.sharepoint.com/Pages/Clinical-Research.aspx
The Clinical Research Program	http://www2.massgeneral.org/crp/
The Harvard Catalyst	http://catalyst.harvard.edu/

The Yvonne L. Munn Center for Nursing Research (Munn Center; see Chapter 3, "Promoting Nursing Research Through the Yvonne L. Munn Center"), within the Institute of Patient Care (IPC), is a recognized member of the MGH research enterprise and one of 30 research departments at the hospital. The executive director of the IPC (a PhD-prepared nurse) serves as a contributing member of ECOR. Membership on ECOR is interdisciplinary and is represented by physicians, nurses, basic and clinical scientists, educators, administrators, lawyers, and statisticians. Members of the Munn Center also serve on committees within the MGH research enterprise, and the Munn Center is a visible entity on the research enterprise organizational chart. Nursing presence on ECOR and other multidisciplinary committees affords nurses a new opportunity to provide input and guidance to inform research policies, participate in hospital-wide research initiatives and educational opportunities, and stay current with research management policies.

Nursing membership on ECOR increases the visibility of nursing research initiatives among the interdisciplinary members of the MGH research enterprise. In addition, the visibility of nurse researchers within the multidisciplinary environments fosters opportunities for future interdisciplinary collaboration and participation in grant writing and promotes the study and design of research efforts that foster the development of evidence and new knowledge. Importantly, nursing presence within the MGH research infrastructure enhances patient care through the identification and development of hospital-wide research priorities designed to meet our patients' needs at the bedside and beyond. A recent initiative called "Find a Researcher" will include PhD-prepared MGH nurse researchers/scientists in a Partners-wide research directory. This listing will be available to all researchers across disciplines and highlight nursing research areas of interest and a brief bio for each scholar.

Interdisciplinary Opportunities to Enhance Research Development

Several key opportunities are available to nurses to influence nurses' ability to participate within the research enterprise. These include membership in the

Institutional Review Board Membership, the Clinical Research Program (CRP), which offers interdisciplinary research education and consultation, and the Harvard Catalyst initiative.

Institutional Review Board Membership

The Institutional Review Board (IRB) process at MGH is known as the Partners Human Research Committee (PHRC). This committee provides an ethical and scientific review of studies involving human subjects within Partners Healthcare ("Human Research Committee/IRB," n.d.; refer to Table 6.1). The PHRC is an interdisciplinary group consisting of physicians, scientists, nurses, statisticians, social workers, ethicists, pharmacists, clergy, and lawyers from across the Partners enterprise. There have been nurse-led study sections, and many nurses are active reviewers of IRB projects. Similar to other IRBs, PHRC members meet at least monthly to review newly submitted and existing protocols based on guidelines, requirements, and ethical principles mandated by regulatory bodies, including the Federal Drug Administration and the Department of Health and Human Services.

Nursing representation on the IRB enhances both research development and research patient care (Cassidy & Oddi, 1993; Robb, 1981). Serving as a reviewer affords nurses the opportunity to be exposed to a variety of interdisciplinary research protocols, ranging from basic science to clinical research. Through careful review of multiple protocols, nurses become familiar with the research process and related protocols, which benefits them in the following ways:

- Learning about the key factors that impact protection of human subjects and that help ensure the ethical conduct of research.

- Knowing areas of research interest within their respective institution, as well as investigators from other disciplines who may have similar areas of research (which might prove helpful when nurses are seeking interdisciplinary collaborators).

- Exposure to diverse research methods and strategies for study implementation, subject recruitment, data collection, and monitoring.

- Improving grant writing skills and increase awareness of common errors and challenges experienced when writing and submitting research proposals.

IRB membership also provides insight into the peer review process when performed by an interdisciplinary team and can broaden a nurse's perspective on ways that each discipline can enhance protocol development and study outcomes.

Nurse membership on the IRB also positively impacts the care of clinical research patients. Nurses are able to offer a seasoned perspective on both physiologic and behavioral aspects of clinical trials and provide a critical assessment of study feasibility (including an evaluation of psycho-social barriers to study participation) and expertise in ethics and the protection of human subjects. In addition, a clinical research nurse's knowledge of the patient and identification of potential conflicts during the administration of a protocol allows these issues to be addressed and changes made to protect the patient engaged in the research experience.

Interdisciplinary Research Education and Consultation

The Clinical Research Program (CRP) at MGH provides a variety of research support, development, and educational services to members of the research community ("About the Clinical Research Program," n.d.; refer to Table 6.1). Nurse researchers have access to consultation services, including study design and implementation, statistical support, and IRB consultation. Specifically, nurse researchers have the opportunity to meet with physicians, scientists, and statisticians for consultation on numerous areas of research, including clinical effectiveness research, patient center outcomes research, translational science, genetics and genomics, and operational evaluations. Nurse researchers have up to 6 hours of free consultation for each scientist to discuss statistical analysis or review a methodological approach to inform a study design. The Munn Center also supports additional time to advance a clinical investigation with CRP consultants and nurse researchers. A part-time, per diem statistician is also available in the Munn Center to work with nurse researchers and clinicians within MGH.

The CRP offers a number of research educational opportunities for clinical investigators, study coordinators, and research nurses on a regular basis. Course instructors are from a variety of disciplines: medicine, nursing, basic scientists, and statisticians. Educational opportunities are open to all participants at no cost. These offerings provide educational opportunities that include grant and manuscript development, subject recruitment, study implementation, research design and methods, as well as inclusion of regulatory updates. Additionally, the CRP provides instruction on the use of the Research Patient Data Registry (RPDR), a Partners clinical data repository for study use with IRB approval ("About the Clinical Research Program," n.d.) and the **R**esearch **S**tudy **V**olunteer **P**rogram, a database of individuals interested in participating in clinical studies (helpful for study recruitment).

The CRP is a resource-rich program that offers nurses at all levels of research expertise the support and education needed for the development of successful research proposals and safe study implementation. Importantly, the interdisciplinary education and consultation available through the CRP allows for sharing of ideas and perspectives across disciplines that is critical for enriching research proposals and meeting the comprehensive needs of our patients.

The Harvard Catalyst and Translational Science Center

The Harvard Clinical and Translational Science Center (CTSC) provides researchers from over 30 collaborating institutions (including MGH) with educational programs, biostatistics consultation, pilot funding, and tools for data collection and research collaboration ("About Harvard Catalyst," n.d.; refer to Table 6.1). Research core facilities, including laboratory services and the Harvard Catalyst Clinical Research Center (HCCRC) are sponsored resources available to all research investigators within the Partners enterprise. The HCCRC at MGH provides comprehensive clinical services from nursing and bio nutrition.

Research nurses on the HCCRC provide direct patient care and assist with the implementation of study procedures with human subjects. Importantly, nurses collaborate with interdisciplinary study teams to carefully review study protocols to ensure human subject safety and adherence to federal research regulations. Nurses at MGH have served as members of grant review panels for the Harvard Catalyst research initiatives, and the nursing director of the HCCRC attends quarterly meetings at the Munn Center to inform the center of opportunities and updates available to the MGH nursing research community. Research nurses from the HCCRC are also members of the IRB and provide critical evaluation and perspective on research subject safety and study feasibility.

Visibility of Nursing Research in a Multidisciplinary Organization

Several opportunities are available for nursing scholars to disseminate the result of clinical inquiry across the MGH community. One is Nursing Research Day, another is Nursing Research Grand Rounds, and the final one discussed in this chapter is Clinical Research Day. These initiatives help promote a community of scholars within nursing and across disciplines.

Nursing Research Day

Nursing Research Day is held each year during Nurse Recognition Week at MGH to showcase nursing research efforts and evidence-based practice projects. Preparing for this event is a year-long effort and reflects research efforts at all levels of nursing. Staff and research scholars work to prepare an agenda that will reflect the broad range of ongoing research activities at MGH. Preparation for the event is initially coordinated by the Munn Center staff. Nurse scientists and researchers within MGH and external faculty nurse scientists assist with the preparation of abstracts, serve on selection committees and work with former and future staff nurses preparing grant applications for the Yvonne L. Munn Research Awards. They also serve on a variety of committees that work throughout the year to present the outcome of various research and evidence-based practice initiatives.

The annual Research Day includes an interactive poster session, presentation of the Yvonne L. Munn Nursing Research Awards (see Chapter 3), and the annual Munn Nursing Research Lecture, presented by a global, esteemed nurse scholar from within or outside of MGH ("Overview of Nursing Research Day," n.d.). This day-long forum allows nurses and other disciplines to engage in dialogue around advancing nursing science and practice with other researchers and national scholars.

THE PREPARATION PROCESS

Nurses from across multiple hospital settings sites are openly invited to submit abstracts for review. Abstract categories include original research, evidenced-based practice, and quality-improvement projects. Abstracts are reviewed by a team of nurse scientists within MGH. The group provides feedback to submitters when needed. Posters are developed by the abstract submitter and printed at the hospital. They are placed on display prior to and following Research Day in prominent locations of MGH for viewing by nurses, other disciplines, the MGH community at large, as well as patients and families.

Posters are evaluated by a team of doctorally prepared nurses on Nursing Research Day, and awards are presented for each abstract category. External faculty nurse scientists appointed by the Munn Center are also invited to submit an abstract for review. In 2014, there were 45 nursing posters on display; this level of exposure increases the visibility of nursing research within MGH organization and beyond. In addition, this initiative highlights the important contribution of nursing research and quality-improvement initiatives to enhance patient care. Nursing Research Day activities also inspire and motivate other nurse colleagues to engage in research and establish collaborations for future projects. Many nurses who engage in these activities have returned to school to seek advanced education, and sometimes even doctoral study.

Nursing Research Grand Rounds

The Munn Nursing Research Grand Rounds were founded in 2013 by the staff of the Munn Center and the Institute for Patient Care. This program provides a forum for past recipients of the Munn Nursing Research Awards and the Munn Fellowship in Nursing Research (see Chapter 3), in addition to nurses and research teams engaged in other scholarship, to present their research findings to the MGH community at large. Invitations are sent to other disciplines, such as Medicine, and since its inception, there has been a growing presence of nurse scholars, staff, and disciplines from across the MGH community in attendance.

Nursing Research Grand Rounds occur quarterly and are open to all members of the MGH community. Each presentation is followed by interdisciplinary dialogue and scholarly discourse, with a focus on publication potential and next research opportunities. The inaugural Munn Nursing Research Grand Rounds (2013) focused on a panel presentation celebrating the Connell Nursing Research Scholars (CNRS; see Chapter 3 as well as Chapter 7, "Researching, Mentoring, and Developing Postdoctoral Scholars") and their research accomplishments. During this session, an overview of the CNRS fellowship was provided, and each scholar presented his or her respective program of research. Leadership from MGH Research Management were present at this session, which again helps increase visibility of nursing research and fellowship support offered for doctorally prepared nurses at MGH. Other Munn Nursing Research Grand Rounds sessions included an interdisciplinary research presentation on ethics (Robinson & Courtwright, 2014) and findings from a qualitative study on experiences with endocrine-based oral therapy among women with breast cancer (Flanagan, 2014). The Munn Nursing Research Grand Rounds are videotaped, and presentations will be available on the Munn Center website in the near future.

Clinical Research Day

Clinical Research Day offers an interdisciplinary celebration of clinical research initiatives conducted by many disciplines across the MGH system ("Clinical Research Program," n.d.). All members of the MGH research community are invited to submit abstracts to a review team, and prizes are awarded to the best abstracts presented. Nurses are visible participants in this work and are eligible for the awards presented during the event. This annual event begins with a keynote address, followed by an interactive research poster session. Nurse researchers who serve as principle investigators or co-investigators have presented posters at MGH Clinical Research Day. Additionally, the Munn Center has an information table during the poster session where resources and information about the Munn Center and nursing research initiatives are shared with interdisciplinary presenters and attendees.

Summary

Promoting nursing research within an interdisciplinary organization requires creativity, dedication, and importantly, support and encouragement from leadership. A critical first step is the preparation and availability of a cohort of doctorally prepared nurses ready to engage in the conduct of research. This is followed by the identification of research resources that are available to scientists across disciplines within the organization and opportunities for nurse access to these resources and opportunities to be a visible presence at interdisciplinary forums such as monthly research meetings to contribute to the research initiatives. Attendance at organization-wide meetings sponsored by the Research Department is a helpful way to become familiar with research leadership, opportunities, and the research infrastructure of the organization. Meeting with research leadership allows nurses to articulate the value of nursing research in a multidisciplinary organization and present concrete examples of how nursing research can enhance patient care, the healthcare workforce, and cost savings.

Participation in research development programs, including education and regulatory sessions offered within or outside of an organization, helps nurse researchers stay current with updated research methods, funding opportunities, and regulatory mandates. The value of serving as a member of an interdisciplinary grant review panel or institutional review board was discussed in this chapter. Nursing's involvement in these efforts promotes new avenues to discuss the significance of nursing research and relate this work to improved patient care within an organization. It also provides the opportunity to discuss innovative approaches to discovery that can be shared across disciplines.

This chapter examined various strategies to increase the visibility of nursing research in a multidisciplinary organization, including Nursing Research Grand Rounds, Nursing Research Day, and Clinical Research Day. Interdisciplinary research events offer scientists from all disciplines an opportunity to participate in dialogue about future research designs and potential grants. If the magnitude of these opportunities is too large for a particular organization, smaller initiatives can be the start of a journey toward promoting a culture of inquiry and discovery. Hosting an annual or biannual nursing research grand rounds or nursing research journal club and inviting interdisciplinary members from throughout the organization's community are examples of initiatives that can help advance a nursing research agenda. Identifying areas of research interest within nursing and across the organization can provide a foundation for growth and development of future nursing research and the identification of collaborative opportunities across an interdisciplinary community.

References

About the clinical research program. (n.d.). Retrieved from http://www2.massgeneral.org/crp/aboutus.html

About Harvard Catalyst. (n.d.). Retrieved from http://catalyst.harvard.edu/about/

Cassidy, V. R., & Oddi, L. F. (1993). Nurses on hospital IRBs: A critical voice in protecting human subjects. *Nursingconnections, 6*(1), 31-38.

Clinical research program. (n.d.). Retrieved from http://www2.massgeneral.org/crp/CR2014_CFA.html

Executive Committee on Research (ECOR). Retrieved from http://ecor.mgh.harvard.edu/default.aspx?node_id=4.

Facts at a glance. Retrieved from http://www.massgeneral.org/research/about/facts.aspx

Flanagan, J. M. (2014, April). Women's experiences of transitioning to endocrine-based oral therapy. Presentation conducted at Massachusetts General Hospital, Boston, MA.

Human research committee/IRB. (n.d.). Retrieved from https://partnershealthcare-public.sharepoint.com/Pages/Clinical-Research.aspx

Overview and history. (n.d.). Retrieved from http://www.massgeneral.org/research/about/overview.aspx

Overview of nursing research day. (n.d). Retrieved from http://www.mghpcs.org/MunnCenter/Research_Day_Overview.asp

Robb, S. S. (1981). Nurse involvement in Institutional Review Boards: The service setting perspective. *Nursing Research, 30*(1), 27-29.

Robinson, E. M., & Courtwright, A. (2014, January). MGH optimum care consultations: descriptive analyses and trends from 2007–2013. Presentation conducted at Massachusetts General Hospital, Boston, MA.

Chapter 7
Researching, Mentoring, and Developing Postdoctoral Scholars

–Dorothy A. Jones, EdD, RN, FAAN, FNI
–Jane M. Flanagan, PhD, ANP-BC

The development of a research agenda within a clinical practice setting requires concentrated time and development of nurses actively engaged in the care of patients. Unlike the academic setting, nurses in practice settings have as their primary focus the care of patients and their families during times of crisis and recovery. The complexity of clinical practices, along with demands linked to the delivery of high-quality, safe, cost-effective, patient-centric, relationship-based quality care, and the coordination of services often limit time nurses have to participate in the conduct of research. Original research initiatives, along with the introduction of evidence-based practice (EBP) projects and quality improvement initiatives, all contribute to the way nurses develop, use, evaluate, and translate research into practice. Each initiative requires leadership and mentoring to advance a nursing research agenda and promote a culture of inquiry.

Little has been written to guide the research mentorship experience of staff nurses as well as the newly prepared postdoctoral individual. This chapter fills that gap by:

- Exploring developments surrounding research mentoring for all nurses to participate in advancing a research agenda in practice.

- Focusing on the importance of mentoring of doctorally prepared nurses. Addressing the challenges related to initiating a career as an independent researcher.

- Discussing the characteristics of good mentoring and core competencies of the mentored research experience as described by the National Postdoctoral Association (NPA) and the National Institutes of Health (NIH) strategies to address postdoctoral mentoring.

- Providing guidelines for a successful postdoctoral mentoring within an academic medical center.

Mentoring and Nursing Staff

Mentoring is a dynamic process used to communicate information to someone else, share knowledge that can help prepare and develop an individual for a new experience, and assist in the creation of a new role. "Mentors help provide a 'safe space' where the expertise, commitment and knowledge of more seasoned professionals can assist nurses to move from 'novice to expert' leaders in patient care or academic excellence" (Banister & Gennaro, 3013, p. 197).

Research Mentoring Opportunities

The Yvonne L. Munn Center for Nursing Research (Munn Center) serves as a catalyst for advancing nursing research throughout the Department of Patient Care Services (PCS) and the Massachusetts General Hospital (MGH) enterprise. Multiple continuing education offerings are available to staff during the year, in addition to individual classes on aspects of research related to the development of research questions, reviewing the literature, generating hypotheses, and developing a research design. Significant opportunities exist within the Munn Center and through participation on committees led by doctorally prepared nurses to develop abstracts or prepare a poster, for example. These learning opportunities enhance staff knowledge and develop expertise in various aspects of the research process. Exposure to these experiences is often the stimulus for many nurses to advance their education and become more active in research activities.

The mentoring opportunities available for MGH nursing staff include the following:

- **Abstract development:** Sessions are regularly held for staff nurses prior to abstract submissions for internal awards. Classes are run by the Munn Center and related committees. Guidelines for abstract submission are reviewed, with clarification related to the development of abstracts for original research, EBP, and quality improvement projects.

- **Educational programming research methods and design:** Offerings from the Munn Center and within the MGH research enterprise are open to staff and members of the Executive Committee on Research (ECOR) community. These programs cover Statistical Package for the Social Sciences (SPSS) and related statistical analysis tools and methodologies (qualitative and quantitative). In addition to accessing computers in the Munn Center, staff can also access computers in a classroom laboratory for direct teaching. Additional SPSS sites are managed by the Munn Center and on the network so that staff members can have SPSS on their desktop for a sustained period of time to review data with a mentor.

- **Evidence-based practice (EBP):** The Munn Center has worked to mentor groups around the implementation of EBP into clinical settings. One example of this was the mentoring of clinical nurse specialists (CNS) to expand their knowledge of EBP and facilitate the development of EBP projects in practice. This was accomplished through a grant from the Health Resources and Services Administration (HRSA) over a 4-year period.

- **Awards supported through the Munn Center:** These awards include a mentoring component. For example the Munn awards for staff nurses include classes and mentored experiences with doctorally prepared nurses, from the time an application is submitted until the final presentation and dissemination of the study.

- **The Munn pre/postdoctoral research awards:** Internal funding is available for doctorally prepared nurses to develop a pilot study or complete a publication. The work is done under the auspices of the Munn Center. The award committee is chaired by doctorally prepared nurses.

- **CNS research task force:** The CNS research task force works with a doctoral mentor from the Munn Center to generate research questions, conduct studies and share findings. For example the CNS research task force was interested in identifying common nursing diagnoses across practice sites and staff preparation to manage the problems. The group, with mentoring from the Munn Center, obtained a grant from NANDA International Foundation to fund the study. Results were disseminated internationally and helped to inform documentation and future educational programs.

- **Doctoral Forum:** Regular meeting of all doctorally prepared nurses at MGH and within PCS, including PhD- and DNP-prepared nurses, are held to promote a culture of inquiry and share research expertise. Monthly meetings are sponsored by the Munn Center. Activities include coaching, mentoring, publication, and grant application reviews, as well as presentations by nurse scholars and funded researchers.

Other mentoring opportunities are also available through the MGH Partners Research Council and related education programs.

Postdoctoral Research Development

The National Institutes of Health (NIH) defines a postdoctoral scholar as "an individual who has received a doctoral degree (or equivalent) and is engaged in a temporary and defined period of mentored advanced training to enhance the professional skills and research independence needed to pursue his or her chosen career path" (NIH Office of Extramural Research, 2011). This rightly assumes that doctoral studies alone do not prepare graduates of doctoral programs to be independent investigators, new academics, or leaders. Rather, they are prepared to launch a new career and, as a result, require significant mentoring.

Research-Intensive Doctoral Preparation

Doctoral education is an immersive experience that launches the graduate as an independent investigator. At the completion of a research-intensive doctoral program, a graduate has at a minimum completed advanced graduate-level coursework, participated in a comprehensive examination, and completed research activities (for example, a pilot study) and defended a dissertation.

Generally within universities, faculty engaged as student mentors for either a research-intensive or practice doctorate derive from time-tenured faculty with the rank of full or associate professor (Gardner & Barnes, 2014). Much has been written in terms of the faculty shortage for preparing bedside nurses and ways to fill this void, but few alternatives address the preparation for research-intensive doctorates in nursing.

Reports indicate that the field of allied health profession that includes nursing has experienced the largest growth in doctoral degrees. From 2007 to 2012, the field of health sciences has experienced the largest increase in both annual enrollments (10.5%) and degrees granted annually (22.6%) as compared to other fields for which a doctorate is awarded (Gonzales, Allum, & Sowell, 2013). Undoubtedly, some of this increase in enrollment and degrees is due in part to the practice doctorate in nursing as well as other health professions as opposed to research doctorates. In either case, the student requires mentoring.

According to American Association of Colleges of Nursing, the average age of full professors and associate professors in nursing is 61.5 and 57.5 years of age, respectively, and together they constitute a mere 28.4% of the faculty with schools of nursing (Fang, Li, & Bednash, 2013). Reports on faculty statistics indicate that the health professions have the lowest number (19.1%) of full-time tenured full professors (College and University Professional Association for

Human Resources, 2103), and more specifically, nursing has 10.5% of its faculty at the rank of tenured full professor and 17.9% at the rank of tenured full-time associate professor (Fang et al., 2013). This increase in demand is simultaneously occurring at a time when funding for all NIH institutes has decreased to historically low numbers.

Fostering Postdoctoral Research: Additional Challenges

Additional factors contribute to the lack of research independence upon completion of a doctoral program, including the following:

- There has been a shift in academia from a focus on education and research aimed at knowledge development to a focus on becoming research intensive and reliant on federal research dollars to be financially viable institutions (Arai, Chech, & Chameau, 2007; Oosterlinck, Debackere, & Cielen, 2002). The issue with the latter is its reliance on federal government for funding.

- The increasing challenge of obtaining NIH or other funding to launch a career as an independent researcher during a time that the NIH budget has been cut by 5% (Kuehn, 2014). This lack of available funding is a problem that is stifling the independent research careers for new investigators across all fields and is paradoxically at a time when federal dollars awarded from the NIH serve as a benchmark for success in academic institutions (Kuehn, 2014). This has resulted in many who would choose academic careers turning to other options. In nursing, this is particularly troubling given that the most educated and potentially talented graduates of doctoral programs are turning away from careers in academia where they are judged by the money they are awarded via the traditional NIH grant mechanism. It has led to a term in the popular media describing this generation of young scientists across all fields turning away from academia as the *lost generation* (El-Seyed, 2013).

At the NIH and the National Institute for Nursing Research (NINR), the success rate for all grants is 9.1%, and for new investigators, the success rate is

8.9% (NIH Research Portfolio Online Reporting Tools, 2013). Collectively, this information suggests that there are more demands on a smaller number of faculty available to prepare a larger number of doctorally prepared nurses interested in achieving research independence at a time when there is more competition for historically less NIH funding.

Postdoctoral Research and Mentoring

In addition to the lack of qualified/seasoned faculty within doctoral programs, opportunities for creating mentoring opportunities for doctoral students are less than ideal. Some programs limit the number and type of student admitted to those who closely match faculty areas of research (Gardner & Barnes, 2014). With decreased funding opportunities available for faculty, there are fewer faculty available with research expertise to mentor doctoral students and advance nursing research opportunities as part of their curriculum. Further complicating the mentoring relationship are these issues:

- Many faculty members are not or have not been funded by the NIH or other extramural funders. This results in the faculty member flexing their area of focus to adapt to the trends that are seemingly more fundable. In other words, their area of focus is in development. Given the demands in academia for faculty to achieve research funding, it is difficult to focus on others (student mentoring) and their potential success (McAlpine & Amundsen, 2011).

- Most mentors have received no formal training for the role and mentor, whether positive or negative, and therefore they mentor based on their own experience of being mentored (Barnes, 2005).

- The mentoring of doctoral students is time-consuming, yet it is not factored into faculty workload (Gardner & Barnes, 2014, p. 63). Maxwell (2008) suggests these issues, consciously or not, can lead to challenges in the relationship and result in jeopardizing the mentee's success.

Achieving a good fit between mentor and mentee can be challenging even if a student's or staff member's area of research interest matches that of a faculty member's. Even when there is a match new challenges emerge when there is a lack of depth and breadth of experiences available to foster sustainable research independence. Mismatches that occur as a result of these limitations negatively impact the experience for both the mentor and mentee.

Despite all these realities, it is essential that doctorally prepared nurses have a strong mentoring experience as they launch or expand their research career. When new doctorally prepared nurses, exposed to various opportunities and challenges throughout their education, enters the practice environment, they must be evaluated as to their ability to advance a program of research independently. Maxwell (2008) suggests that the best mentors have themselves been mentored well.

Gardner and Barnes (2014) describe the role of the mentor as a guide, a scholar, a colleague, and role model who socializes the individual into the profession, may serve on grant proposals, and guides research and other scholarly work. It has been reported that only 57% of students entering a doctoral program graduate within 10 years (Council on Graduate Education, 2008), and those that do graduate now need a postdoctoral degree to be considered for a new career as an independent investigator and academic.

The recognition of these issues facing the newly prepared doctoral person has accelerated the addition of postdoctoral training or fellowships as a requirement for new investigators to begin a research career. Postdoctoral programs inherently recognize that beginning a demanding new career as an independent investigator is part of a process that takes time and is filled with both successes and failures. This and other challenges place new demands on the clinical settings interested in supporting new and mid-career doctorally prepared nurses seeking to advance a nursing research agenda outside of an academic setting.

Postdoctoral Research in Clinical Practice

The completion of doctoral education is not an endpoint, but rather the commencement of a new career as an independent researcher, leader, and scholar. Without a mentor guiding the way for this new career, the newly prepared doctoral students will not achieve their potential. As a result, the mentoring experience is considered by many to be one of the most important endeavors for both the student or post-doctorally prepared person.

Appropriate mentoring is described by the NIH and examples are shown in Table 7.1. Collectively, these experiences provide postdoctorally prepared persons with opportunities that will help them be competent.

TABLE 7.1 Examples of Mentoring Opportunities for Nursing Staff at the Munn Center

ROLE	MENTORING OPPORTUNITIES
Staff nurses	Seek mentoring from Munn Center and doctoral staff to identify researchable topics, clinical questions, and related research titles needed to conduct clinical inquiry.
	Participate actively in relevant Collaborative Governance Committees and EBP initiatives.
	Participate in ongoing mentoring to support staff nurses' active participation in research initiatives (e.g., the mentored Munn Awards, EBP and quality improvement projects).
Master's-prepared nurses	Participate in mentoring Collaborative Governance Committees and EBP work initiatives. (For example, CNSs are active co-investigators in an HRSA-funded project.) Seek mentoring by more senior researchers to advance one's own research and begin to publish.
	Members of a research team: To participate in grant proposal with doctorally prepared principal investigator (PI) (e.g., Clinical Nurse Specialist Research Task Force).
Master's and doctoral students	Participate as a research assistant/data collector in Munn Center-funded projects (mentored by a PI).
	Identify practicum experience and seek mentoring from a nurse scientist at the MGH.
	Participate in mentor's publications.

continues

TABLE 7.1 *continued*

ROLE	MENTORING OPPORTUNITIES
Doctorally prepared nurses	Engage in mentored experience as a co-investigator on grant.
	Mentoring opportunities from staff in the Munn Center to advance grant development.
	Serve as a mentor to staff on projects and implementing research.
	Participate in the Doctoral Forum activities and Munn Center research teams
	Apply for mentored experience as a Connell Nursing Research Scholar.
	Apply for a Munn Pre/Post-Mentoring Award.

The mentoring opportunities described in the preceding table are essential experiences that contribute to the development and advancement of an independent investigator and burgeoning scholar. The NPA specifies that the goal of the postdoctorate experience is not mere exposure, but rather competence. They use a definition of competency and describe it as being a skill that is acquired through being able to consistently demonstrate a high level of performance (in this case, skills related to a career in research) (NPA, 2010).

The following are recommended goals of ongoing mentorship pre-post doctorate (NIH, 2013; NPA, 2010):

- Opportunity to work collaboratively on the research of an experienced faculty member

- Preparing materials, including abstracts, posters, or papers for conference presentations

- Publishing a scholarly article in a peer-reviewed journal either as a single author or in conjunction with a faculty member

- Assuming responsibilities congruent with the career for which they are being prepared (e.g., teaching experiences for an academic career)

- Socializing with other scholars in the field

Postdoctoral Mentor-Mentee Relationship

The mentor-mentee relationship is a critically important one in terms of career development, researcher independence, and leadership. Until recently, however, there were few, if any, guidelines for postdoctoral mentoring. As a result of the challenges related to the mentorship experience, the NIH (2013) now calls for institutions to develop and report to the NIH the individual development plans (IDPs) for each NIH-supported graduate student, fellow, or postdoctoral candidate. These IDPs are to be broad in nature, but the goal of the IDP is to prepare the individual to reach his or her career goals and independently contribute to ongoing science development.

Much of what the NIH (2013) calls for is captured by the NPA's (2010) six core competencies for postdoctoral training. The six core competencies are as follows:

- Discipline-specific conceptual knowledge

- Research skill development

- Communication skills

- Professionalism

- Leadership and management skills

- Responsible conduct of research

The NPA (2010) suggests that while some of these competencies may have been gained during graduate study, the individual pursuing the postdoctorate should use these as criteria to evaluate the mentor and the program. It also suggests that the potential postdoctoral individual complete a self-evaluation of skills initially and on an ongoing basis with the mentor to evaluate growth, maintain dialogue, and determine areas of weakness and whether the competencies are being met. Using the competency checklist, the individual rates him or herself on a scale of 1 (needs attention) to 9 (extremely competent). NPA (2010) checklist includes this list of competencies.

- Discipline-Specific Conceptual Knowledge
  - Analytical Approach to Defining Scientific Questions
  - Design of Scientifically Testable Hypotheses
  - Broad-Based Knowledge Acquisition
  - Interpretation and Analysis of Data
- Professional/Research Skill Development
  - Literature Search Strategies and Effective Interpretation
  - Experimental Design
  - Statistical Analysis
  - Data Analysis and Interpretation
  - Laboratory Techniques and Safety
  - Principles of the Peer Review Process
- Communication Skills
  - Writing
  - Speaking
  - Teaching
  - Interpersonal
  - Special Situations
- Professionalism
  - Workplace
  - Institutional

- Collegial

- Universal

- Leadership and Management Skills

  - Leadership-Strategic Vision

  - Leadership-Motivating and Inspiring Others

  - Management-Project Management

  - Management-Data and Resource Management

  - Management-Research Staff Management

- Responsible Conduct of Research

  - Conflicts of Interest

  - Data Ownership and Sharing

  - Publication Practices and Responsible Authorship

  - Identifying and Mitigating Research Misconduct

  - Research with Human Subjects (when applicable)

  - Research Involving Animals (when applicable)

Even with the advent of these important guidelines, it is worth noting that many describe the relationship between the mentor and mentee as a reciprocal one (Barnes, 2005; Barnes & Austin, 2009; Gardner & Barnes, 2014; Maxwell, 2008; NPA, 2010). The NPA (2010) does suggest the mentor and mentee both use this self-evaluation, but it is the mentee and his or her progress that is evaluated. Inherent to some philosophies of education, it is pedagogically sound for the mentor and mentee relationship to be one in which each will learn from one another (Boston College, 2003). To have a truly successful relationship, the mentor and mentee must be able to openly dialogue about the experience and ways each person contributes. This involves a process of discernment and self-reflection for both the mentor and mentee so that each can grow from the experience. Maxwell (2008) discusses this notion and states that to truly develop leaders it is imperative that mentors recognize their own inner feelings as they mentor. He also suggests that by reflecting, mentors may recognize their own need for mentoring. This iterative process of reflecting and seeking new skills for all involved in the mentoring process creates leaders ready to lead.

Connell Nursing Research Postdoctoral Scholars

The Connell Nursing Research Scholars (CNRS) program at the MGH was introduced to the Munn Center in 2012 through the generous and visionary support of the Connell family. The program is designed to address the development of a growing number of nurse scholars who achieved the research doctorate and remain in a clinical practice setting. Given the challenges discussed earlier in this chapter, there is a need to develop these scholars by providing new opportunities for mentoring and scholarship. The development and experiences of mentoring are core aspects of the CNRS.

The CNRS program provides nurse researchers with the time and mentoring to advance multidisciplinary patient- and family-centered care through nursing research (Jones, 2012, p. 11). As doctorally prepared nurse researchers actively engage in the care of patients and families within the practice setting, the CNRS funding offers selected scholars the time to advance a program of research, addresses the strategic goals of PCS, and develop focal areas of nursing research within MGH and beyond. As of this writing, 9 of the more than 50 doctorally prepared nurses at the MGH have been named Connell Nursing Research Scholars. Their research, supported by philanthropic funding from the Connell family, has helped promote nursing research in several important areas of national, if not global, concern.

CNRS Program Objectives

The goals of the CNRS program are designed to provide guidance to the scholars and support the research goals of the scholars and their mentors. Applicants to the CNRS program are asked to address five program objectives in their proposed research plan:

- Developing knowledge to advance patient care through research that includes designing a plan and timeline to reach goals and participate in regular meetings with internal program advisor and external mentor

- Becoming proficient in the conduct of research within the clinical practice environment, reviewing grant guidelines with mentor, and submitting applications for external funding

- Becoming an active participant in the facilitation and translation of nursing research into practice and in collaboration with teams at MGH

- Participating in forums at MGH and beyond to disseminate research findings

- Continuing to work with mentors to network and collaborate around areas of research importance to nursing and patient care

CNRS Application Process

A formal application process is available from the Munn Center website for potential CNRS candidates to review and complete online. Applicants early in their postdoctoral career as well as mid-career nurse researchers with an established program of research are eligible to apply. Each applicant addresses a series of demographic questions and then answers questions that include describing how the CNRS program will help advance research interests and contribute to advancing goals of PCS and MGH.

Prior to submitting an application, all submissions must be reviewed with the candidates' supervisor. This is essential so that the leadership is informed and supports the time allocated for research at the unit or department level. The completed application includes:

- Project name

- A proposed weekly and overall timeline

- A potential nationally known mentor in the area of research identified by the applicant

- A current curriculum vitae (CV), including past publications and funding

All applications are submitted to the Munn Center and reviewed by advisory board with members from MGH nursing and other disciplines as well as external experts from the nursing community. CNRS scholars are announced to the community and the Connell family.

CNRS Mentoring Experience

The CNRS program offers scholars a mentoring experience to help advance their research career. Two nurse scientists (currently Diane L. Carroll and Dorothy A. Jones) within the Munn Center help to facilitate the program from application to implementation and evaluation. They meet individually with each CNRS throughout the year of the award and hold regularly scheduled meetings with all scholars to discuss project implementation and address challenges. These nurse scientists help coordinate mentor visits to MGH and the CNRS travel to mentor sites. The ultimate outcome of the CNRS award is the submission of an external grant for funding and publications as well as national and international presentations.

In addition to the support provided to the CNRSs by the Munn Center staff, each CNRS identifies a nationally known nurse scholar to enhance the post-doctoral experience. The mentor, called a program advisor, is described as "a visionary nurse leader and experienced researcher with a demonstrated ability to advance a research agenda especially within a clinical practice environment" (Connell Nursing Research Scholars Program, 2014).

The mentor and mentee build a research development plan and identify ways that they can work collaboratively to enhance research competence in areas of shared research concentration. The individual works with the mentor to prepare abstracts, write grants, and disseminate research. The mentor collaborates with the mentee on projects and engages the mentee in networking activities and research activities. All CNRS scholars are expected to publish alone or with their mentor and to work to achieve the goals of their development plan.

The CNRS program leaders meet with the scholar on a regular basis. The scholar's external mentor is expected to attend at least one onsite meeting where the mentor meets the scholar, leaders at the clinical site, other doctorally prepared nurses (individually and one on one) and presents a paper to a multi-disciplinary audience that is then disseminated on the Munn website. To date, distinguished CNRS mentors have included Patricia Stone, PhD, RN, FAAN, Angela Barron McBride, PhD, RN, FAAN, Mary Sullivan, PhD, RN, FAAN, Linda Aiken, PhD, RN, FAAN, FRCN, Jean Watson, PhD, RN, ANH-BC, FAAN, Martha Curley, PhD, RN, FAAN, and Ardith Doorenbos, PhD, RN, FAAN.

The CNRS scholars also have access to the MGH Research Center for additional help with biostatistics and research design. External faculty nurse scientists appointed to the Munn Center are also available to collaborate with scholars and assist with discussions to advance the science.

CNRS Research Foci

Clearly identified areas of research concentration developed by the CNRS researcher have emerged over time and continue to grow.

The list of the areas of research concentration under inquiry as of this writing are as follows:

- Workforce Evaluation and Leadership Influence over the Professional Practice Environment (Development and Testing of the Leadership Influence over the Professional Practice Environment Scale – LIPPES)

- Expanding Knowledge Needed to Enhance Effective Pain Management (Chronic Pain Management and Persistent Pain Management in Older Adults)

- Infant Feeding and the Newborn Intensive Care Special Care Nursery (Infant-Driven Feeding Assessment Tool)

- Care of the Elderly and Palliative Care (HRSA-funded follow-up to the AgeWise educational program)

- Expansion of Oral Care Interventions for Critically Ill Patients

- Health of Vulnerable Populations: Woman's Health and Menopause in HIV-Infected Women

- Relationship-Based Care: Knowing the Patient and Complementary Healing Practices

- Reduction of Hospital Acquired Infections (CAUTI)

It is interesting to note that these areas of research concentration are similar to the research within PCS overall (see Chapter 3, "Promoting Nursing Research Through the Yvonne L. Munn Center").

CNRS Postdoctoral Program Outcomes

Since the inception of the CNRS program, there have been many outcomes to advance the research careers of the scholars, including the following

- Over 35 publications in high-impact journals (e.g., *Journal of Gerontology Nursing, Journal of Nursing Administration, Clinical Orthopedics and Related Research*, and *Menopause*)

- 30 presentations at national and international meetings (NANDA International, the North American Menopause Society, the American Academy of Pain Management, and Sigma Theta Tau International)

- 10 grant submissions, with several grants funded, for example, the American Nurses Foundation, Tri Service Nursing Camp Grant and a 5-year extension of an NIH Perioperative Cognitive Behavioral Pain Management Center of Excellence on Pain Education (Co EPE).

In addition, there have been significant professional achievements, including the following:

- Selection as a Robert Wood Johnson Fellow

- Appointments as visiting professor to MIT and Boston College

- Promotion to assistant professor at Harvard Medical School

- Appointments to editorial boards

- An appointment as a Watson Scholar

CNRS Follow-Up

Continued appointments of Connell Nursing Researh Scholars are occurring on a regular basis—the most recent, as of this writing, in January of 2015. In addition, four Connell Competitive Grants were recently announced for CNRS scholars who are still analyzing data from their original awards. Also, all previous and current CNRS scholars meet on a regular basis to discuss their research development plan and next steps for grant submissions and publications. Many are still in contact with their mentors. The CNRS scholars see themselves as mentors to staff, working to engage them in grant writing and research opportunities as they move their work forward. The Munn Center leadership continues to monitor and oversee implementation of the Connell Scholars program. The center's director attends meetings of the Connell Nursing Research Scholars Group; the scholars who have participated in the CNRS program to promote their own work seek to initiate new research and initiate larger research initiatives across MGH. Several CNRS scholars are pursuing multidisciplinary research opportunities and funding (e.g., Patient-Centered Outcomes Research Institute [PCORI] grants and participation in the MGH Research Council).

Summary

Advancing a nursing research agenda within a clinical practice environment requires personnel, resources, and a commitment by nursing and organizational leadership as to the important impact nursing inquiry can have on patient care. Philanthropic support, development of research partnerships, and internal and external funding, along with a plan to advance nursing scholarship and clinical investigation, can have a dramatic impact on staff satisfaction and professional development of clinicians.

References

Arai, K. I., Chech, T., & Chameau, J. L. (2007). The future of research universities. *EMBO Reports*, *8*(9), 804–810.

Banister, G., & Gennaro, S. (2013). Mentorship and best practices for mentorship. In Ives Erickson, J., Jones, D., & Ditomassi, M. *Fostering care at the bedside: Professional practice for the bedside leader from Massachusetts General Hospital*. Indianapolis, IN: Sigma Theta Tau International, 196-217.

Barnes, B. J. (2005). *Success in graduate school: How exemplary advisors guide their doctoral advisees.* (Unpublished doctoral dissertation.) Doctoral dissertation, Michigan State University, Department of Education Administration.

Barnes, B. J., & Austin, A. E. (2009). The role of doctoral advisors: A look at advising from the advisor's perspective. *Innovative Higher Education, 33(5),* 297-315.

Boston College. (2003). A pocket guide to jesuit education. Retrieved from http://www.bc.edu/content/bc/offices/mission/publications/guide.html

College and University Professional Association for Human Resources (2103). Faculty in higher education salary survey for the 2012-2013 academic year. Retrieved from http://www.cupahr.org/surveys/files/salary2013/FHE4-2013-Executive- Summary.pdf

Connell Nursing Research Scholars Program. (2014). Retrieved from http://www.mghpcs.org/munncenter

Council of Graduate Education. (2008). Ph.D. completion and attrition: Analysis of the baseline program data from the Ph.D. completion project. Washington, DC: Author.

El-Seyed, A. (2013). The sequester and the "Lost Generation" in health research: How it could rob our future of important advancements. *The 2x2 project: Health behind the headlines.* Retrieved from http://the2x2project.org/a-lost-generation-in-health-science/

Fang, D., Li, Y., & Bednash, G. D. (2013). *2012-2013 Salaries of instructional and administrative nursing faculty in baccalaureate and graduate programs in nursing.* Washington, DC: American Association of Colleges of Nursing.

Gardner, S.K., & Barnes, B. J., (2104). Advising and mentoring doctoral students: A Handbook. *University of Maine Faculty Monographs.* Book 210. Retrieved from http://digitalcommons.library.umaine.edu/fac_monographs/210

Gonzales, L. M., Allum, J. R., & Sowell, R. S. (2013). *Graduate enrollment and degrees: 2002 to 2012.* Washington, DC: Council of Graduate Schools.

Kuehn, B. M. (2014). Budget woes, sequester place researchers in a bind: Young researchers hard hit. *JAMA, 311(1),* 15-16.

Jones, D. (2012). Patient Care Services, Massachusetts General Hospital. *Caring Headlines,* December.

Maxwell, J. (2008). *Mentoring 101: What every leader needs to know.* Thomas Nelson Inc.

McAlpine, L., & Amundsen, C. (Eds.) (2011). Doctoral Education: Research-Based Strategies for Doctoral Students, Supervisors, and Administrators. London, Springer.

National Institutes of Health (NIH). (2013). NIH encourages institutions to develop individual development plans for graduate students and postdoctoral researchers. Retrieved from: http://grants.nih.gov/grants/guide/notice-files/NOT-OD-13-093.html

National Postdoctoral Association (NPA). (2010). The NPA postdoctoral core competencies toolkit. Retrieved from http://www.nationalpostdoc.org/competencies

(NIH) Office of Extramural Research (2011). Frequently asked questions NRSA research training. Retrieved from http://grants.nih.gov/training/q&a.htm#2491

NIH Research Portfolio Online Reporting Tools (RePORT). (2013). Research project success rates for the selected institute. Retrieved from http://www.report.nih.gov/success_rates/Success_ByIC_Details.cfm?IC=NINR&FY=2013

Oosterlinck, A., Debackere, K., & Cielen, G. (2002). Balancing basic and applied research. *EMBO Reports,* 3(1), 2-5.

Chapter 8
Evaluating Professional Practice in Nursing Research

–Mary E. Duffy, PhD, RN, FAAN

After the publication of the first Magnet® hospital study (McClure, Poulin, Souvin, & Wandelt, 1983), professional practice models have become increasingly important in today's healthcare settings. Ives Erickson and Ditomassi (2011) define a professional practice model as a well-designed framework that permits nurses to clearly articulate contributions to practice from the profession. The Massachusetts General Hospital (MGH) Professional Practice Model (PPM), formulated in 1996 and revised in 2006, incorporates the major findings from the first Magnet hospital study: nurse autonomy in clinical practice, control over practice, collaborative relationships with physicians, as well as other elements derived from extant organizational and nursing research (Ives Erickson & Ditomassi, 2011). At MGH, the PPM represents Patient Care Services staff commitment to delivering seamless and knowledge-based high-quality care to patients and their families (Ives Erickson, 2012).

The purpose of this chapter is to:

- Detail the development of the MGH PPM and its major elements

- Describe the MGH professional practice environment and the development and psychometric appraisal of multidimensional measures used to evaluate this environment

- Discuss two electronic data collection methods currently used at MGH for PPM evaluation and other health-focused studies: Qualtrics Research Suite and REDCap

- Present an account of other instruments derived from the PPM and Revised Professional Practice Environment (RPPE) scale

- List specific research studies completed around the world springing from the PPM and/or instruments generated by MGH nurse researchers

MGH Professional Practice Models

Following the development of a comprehensive strategic plan, the first MGH PPM was created in 1996 and delineated the work and contributions made by nurses and other health professionals across various settings and levels of care within the hospital. According to Ives Erickson (2000), the MGH PPM served to:

- Articulate the work of clinicians across a variety of settings

- Provide a framework to guide clinical practice, education, research, and administration

- Promote communication among disciplines and between clinicians and the organization

- Guide the allocation of resources

- Provide a framework for the evaluation of clinical practice and serve as a marketing tool both internally and externally

Subsequent revisions to this PPM were made in both 2006 and 2014.

MGH PPM: 1996

In recent publications, Ives Erickson and Ditomassi (Ives Erickson & Ditomassi, 2011; Ives Erickson, 2012) define the major components of the original 1996 model as follows:

- **Philosophy:** A statement derived from the values, principles, and beliefs held by nursing and other healthcare disciplines that comprise the MGH Patient Care Services. The philosophy includes each discipline's beliefs, values, and contributions. Nursing's philosophy focuses on patient care, education, research, and the contributions nurses make to promote quality and safety in care delivery.

- **Standards of practice:** Defined as the practice application of values and philosophy whose purpose is to safeguard the highest quality of care for all patients by all providers regardless of their experience level.

- **Collaborative decision-making/governance:** A decision-making process built on teamwork and team learning that empowers clinicians with the authority, responsibility, and accountability for patient care. Successful collaborative governance ensures that clinicians control their own practice, acknowledge each caregiver discipline's contribution, and incorporate them into healthcare delivery.

- **Professional development:** Activities designed to ensure that nurses at all levels provide high-quality care to patients. These activities include enhancing nurses' leadership skills, professional growth, and career advancement.

- **Patient care delivery model:** Defined and designed to promote the delivery of the highest quality of cost-effective, patient-centric care.

- **Privileging, credentialing, and peer review:** Processes designed to ensure that patients and their families receive the highest quality of care from nurses and other providers who possess the appropriate credentials for licensure, certification, and competency-based training. Peer review supports nurses' autonomy and accountability for their practice within the work setting and helps improve individual and organizational performance.

- **Research:** Defined as a spirit of inquiry that, when actualized, produces a systematic body of relevant knowledge that underpins professional clinical practice. Research is an essential aspect of the model that bridges the gap between academic knowledge and theory and clinical practice.

- **Theory-based practice:** Defined as the philosophic, structural, and theoretical foundations of clinical practice, the *whys* of what nurses and other clinical staff do.

MGH Revised PPM: 2006

In 2006, MGH nursing leadership, based on evaluation of the PPM elements, updated the PPM to include the following elements (Ives Erickson & Ditomassi, 2011):

- **Narrative culture:** Verbal/written accounts that permit staff sharing and reflection on clinical practice. Such sharing helps clinicians to see their practice differently, fosters communication and dialogue, and helps them to gain greater understanding of their clinical reasoning and knowledge base. Clinical narratives are the ones that MGH values highly because they provide descriptions of real care and the environments in which it occurred.

- **Clinical recognition and advancement:** The vehicle through which MGH staff acquire, develop, and master specific skills along the novice-to-expert continuum. It is viewed as an effective retention tool at MGH and implemented through the MGH Clinical Recognition Program. The reflective process is central to the program, helping clinicians to understand what shapes their practice and use information meaningfully, thus fostering their professional growth and excellence in caring for patients.

- **Innovation and entrepreneurial teamwork:** Defined as a process for inventing something new or improving on that which already exists (Blakeney, Carleton, McCarthy, & Coakley, 2009). MGH considers this element as critical to creating a professional practice environment that embraces change to make sure that patient care delivery and associated structures meet the healthcare needs of the patients served.

- **Patient-centeredness:** Considered the most critical and central piece of the PPM, touching all PPM components. To achieve this focus on MGH patients and their families, the component requires resources, programs, and processes that include the six pillars of safety and quality delineated by the Institute of Medicine (IOM) in its 2001 report on creating a new health system for the 21st century, as follows (IOM, 2001):

  - **Efficiency:** Avoiding waste related to equipment, supplies, ideas, and energy.

  - **Safety:** Avoiding injuries to patients from the care is supposed to help them.

  - **Equity:** Providing care that does not vary in quality because of personal characteristics such as ethnicity, gender, geographic region, and socioeconomic status.

  - **Effectiveness:** Providing services based on scientific knowledge to all who could benefit and refraining from providing services to those not likely to benefit (avoiding underuse and overuse).

  - **Timeliness:** Reducing waits and sometimes-harmful delays for those who receive and those who give care.

  - **Patient-centeredness:** Providing care that is respectful of and responsive to individual patient preferences, needs, and values and ensuring that patient values guide all clinical decisions.

MGH Revised PPM: 2014

At an annual executive team retreat in September 2014, feedback about the PPM was reviewed, and the following three changes were made:

- **Professional development was expanded to include lifelong learning:** The concept of lifelong learning was added to the professional development component to highlight that learning is an ongoing process.

- **Research was expanded to include evidence-based practice (EBP):** In addition to the definition, EBP is defined as the conscientious use/integration of the best research evidence with clinical expertise and patient preferences in nursing practice (Sackett, Straus, Richardson, Rosenberg, & Haynes, 2000).

- **Patient-centeredness was changed to the concept of relationship-based care (RBC):** RBC is a model and an operational framework that improves safety, quality, patient satisfaction, and staff satisfaction by improving the relationship between caregivers and the patients and families they service, the caregiver's relationship with self, and the relationship among members of the healthcare team (Koloroutis, 2004).

In summary, the evolving MGH PPM serves as a clearly articulated framework with MGH nurses as the most important group for connecting all the model's elements to achieve exemplary clinical outcomes.

The MGH Professional Practice Environment

Since the early 1980s, the clinical practice environment has assumed increasing importance in healthcare delivery. A review of the nursing literature indicates that four major terms are used for this construct:

- Work environment (McClure, Poulin, Sovie, & Wandelt, 1983)

- Practice environment (Lake, 2002)

- Healthy work environment (Sherman & Pross, 2010)

- Professional practice environment (Ives Erickson, 2012)

    The term *professional practice environment* (PPE) is used at MGH to represent the organizational culture that advances the clinical practice of nursing and other health professionals by ensuring unity of purpose, organizational alignment, and collaborative decision-making that is designed to let all MGH staff knowingly participate in change.

Evaluating the MGH PPM Through the SPPPE

Since 1997, the PPM elements have been systematically evaluated internally and externally. The internal evaluation takes place at regular intervals, usually every 12 to 18 months, through the Staff Perceptions of the Professional Practice Environment (SPPPE) survey, given to all MGH Patient Care Services disciplines: Ambulatory Care, Chaplaincy, Child Life Specialists, Nursing, Occupational Therapy, Physical Therapy, Respiratory Therapy, Social Services, and Speech/ Language Pathology. This survey is described in the next section.

The external evaluation consists of applying and securing Magnet® recognition by the American Nurses Credentialing Center, considered the highest evidence that the PPM is alive and thriving in the MGH PPE (Ives Erickson & Ditomassi, 2011). Magnet recognition is discussed in depth in the next chapter.

The SPPPE contains five major components:

- Demographic information about respondents

- The PPE scale (Ives Erickson, Duffy, Gibbons, Fitzmaurice, & Ditomassi, 2004), used from 1997 through 2005, or the Revised PPE (RPPE) scale (Ives Erickson, Duffy, Ditomassi, & Jones, 2009) used from 2007 through 2013

- The Adapted Job Enjoyment scale (Brayfield & Rothe, 1951)

- Nine unidimensional scales, eight of which measure satisfaction with elements of the PPE on a six-point scale from very dissatisfied to very satisfied, and one overall work satisfaction item measured on a four-point scale from very dissatisfied to very satisfied

- An open-ended question offering all clinicians the opportunity to provide additional input and reflections about the PPE at MGH

MGH administrators view the SPPPE evaluation as an effective report card of the health of the MGH PPE. They use SPPPE findings to more fully understand and appreciate those organizational factors that enhance clinical practice and what support structures might be needed to achieve the IOM's six pillars discussed earlier. The last SPPPE evaluation occurred in April, 2015. Exploratory questions focusing on the concept of power as knowing participation in change (Barrett, 1989, 1990; Caroselli & Barrett, 1998b), are being explored.

Development and Evaluation of the PPE Scale

The PPE scale, developed in late 1998 to evaluate the effectiveness of the PPM, initially consisted of 35 items measuring eight PPE elements, as follows:

- Leadership and Autonomy in Clinical Practice (five items) is the quality or state of being self-governing and exercising professional judgment in a timely fashion (Aiken, Sochalski, & Lake, 1997).

- Staff Relationships with Physicians (two items) are those associations with physicians that facilitate exchange of important clinical information (Aiken et al., 1997).

- Control over Practice (six items) signifies sufficient intra-organizational status to influence others and deploy resources when necessary for good patient care (Aiken, Havens, & Sloane, 2000).

- Communication About Patients (three items) is defined as the degree to which a patient's shared information is related promptly to the people who need to be informed through open channels of interchange (Shortell, Rousseau, Gillies, Devers, & Simons, 1991).

- Teamwork (four items) is viewed as a conscious activity aimed at achieving unity of effort in the pursuit of shared objectives (Zimmerman et al., 1993).

- Handling Disagreement and Conflict (eight items) represents the degree to which managing discord is addressed using a problem-solving approach (Zimmerman et al., 1993).

- Internal Work Motivation (four items) is self-generated encouragement completely independent of external factors such as pay, supervision, or co-workers (Hackman & Oldham, 1976, 1980; Ives Erickson, 2000).

- Cultural Sensitivity (three items) is a set of attitudes and practices/policies that respects and accepts cultural differences (Ives Erickson, 2000).

Content validity, along with readability and clarity of items, was established by seven MGH staff members. After minor editing, all items were retained and placed on a four-point Likert scale of SA (strongly agree), A (agree), D (disagree), and SD (strongly disagree). This PPE version was used from 1999 through 2001 to evaluate the effectiveness of the MGH PPE and to determine changes in the environment from year to year.

During these years, seven of the eight PPE subscales demonstrated satisfactory internal consistency reliability coefficients. However, the four-item Internal Work Motivation subscale had less-than-adequate internal consistency ($r^c = 0.63$), most likely due to high homogeneity of staff responses on the items. Therefore, four additional items were developed, content validated, and added to the subscale. Also, one item in the Handling Disagreement/Conflict subscale that contained two ideas was edited to form two items to eliminate possible confusion for respondents. The PPE scale, now 40 items in length, was the version used to determine the psychometric adequacy of the measure.

PPE Scale Psychometric Evaluation

A psychometric evaluation of the PPE scale was undertaken in 2002 with a sample of 849 MGH clinical staff from nursing and other health disciplines. Item-total correlations for the PPE scale demonstrated that 38 of the 40 items were above the 0.30 cutoff for inclusion in the scale (Nunnally & Bernstein, 1994). After dropping these items from the scale, the Cronbach's alpha internal consistency reliability for the now 38-item scale was 0.93 (Ives Erickson et al., 2004).

Principal components analysis (PCA) with Varimax rotation and Kaiser normalization was next computed on the 38-item PPE scale. Although there were nine components with eigenvalues > 1.0, the more parsimonious scree test showed an eight-component solution. Because the scale was designed to measure eight dimensions, a second PCA was performed specifying eight components. All 38 items loaded above the 0.30 loading cutoff on the expected component, confirming the eight-component structure and accounting for 61% of explained variance. Cronbach's alpha internal consistency reliability coefficients ranged from 0.78 to 0.88 on the PPE subscales. So, the 38-item PPE scale was judged reliable and factorially valid for use in subsequent research studies. The full description of the psychometric evidence of the PPE is reported elsewhere (Ives Erickson et al., 2004).

Development and Evaluation of the RPPE Scale

After strategic goals were changed in 2005, the PPE scale underwent revision. Two items, designed to identify where disputes originated, were added to the Handling Disagreement/Conflict subscale. The now 42-item RPPE scale underwent minor editing to provide further clarity. This RPPE scale was then converted to an online survey using Qualtrics, a web-based tool for creating and conducting online surveys. Psychometric evaluation of the online RPPE scale was done on the 2006 SPPPE respondents. Because the sample size was large (N = 1,550), a random-sample cross-validation procedure (Cudeck & Brown, 1983; Fry & Duffy, 2001) was used in the psychometric evaluation of the online RPPE scale. The 1,550 sample was randomly divided into two random samples of 775 respondents each: a calibration sample (CS) and a validation sample (VS). In the cross-validation procedure, the CS (n = 775) was used to derive the underlying PCA component structure; the VS (n = 775) was used to confirm/validate the component structure.

RPPE Scale Psychometric Evaluation

The Cronbach's alpha internal consistency reliability was 0.93 for the CS and 0.92 for the VS.

Despite that the same five items in each sample were below the 0.30 item-total correlation cutoff, all items were kept in the RPPE to determine how well they performed in subsequent PCAs.

Specifying eight components, a PCA with Varimax rotation and Kaiser normalization was next computed on the CS and VS using the 42-item RPPE scale. Inspection of the rotated component matrix demonstrated a parsimonious and interpretable solution in both groups. Of the 42 RPPE items, the same 39 items, with loadings above the 0.30 cutoff level, loaded together to form the expected component in both the CS and VS samples, thus confirming the component structure. These 39 items forming eight component scales accounted for 59.2% of explained variance in the CS and 59.7% variance in the VS. Cronbach's alpha internal consistency reliability coefficients for the eight component subscales ranged from 0.80 to 0.87 in the CS and from 0.81 to 0.88 in the VS. So, the RPPE was judged reliable and valid for use in future research endeavors and demonstrated psychometric equivalence to its predecessor, the PPE scale.

Similarly to the PPM, the instrument is modified to reflect changes in the PPM and psychometrically evaluated when changes are made.

The Use of Web-Based Survey Platforms for PPM Evaluation and Other Health-Focused Research

Until late 2009, MGH conducted SPPPE surveys using paper-pencil, hard copy methods. Gathering data in this fashion was expensive in terms of time and financial resources. Surveys had to be distributed and collected manually. A program had to be written in a statistical database that data entry personnel would then use to manually enter each respondent's survey data. Once done, the data file could be prepared and analyzed to produce descriptive and other statistical results. Finally, a study report would be written based on the statistical analyses. In 2010, MGH moved from conducting surveys using hard copy to two web-based systems, both of which are described in this section.

Qualtrics Research Suite

Since 2010, the SPPPE survey has been developed and implemented via Qualtrics Research Suite (QRS), a user-friendly web-based survey research platform. Because QRS is completely browser-based and requires no software installation on the user's computer, researchers can access it from any location with Internet access. QRS is considered the standard survey and research platform used by universities today, including every major U.S. university and 97 of the top 100 business schools (*EdTech Times* Staff, 2014). MGH has an annual contract with Qualtrics for use of QRS.

Due to its intuitive user interface, rigorous survey design functionality, robust reporting, and analytics capabilities to conduct simple or sophisticated research,

QRS is an extremely flexible platform for conducting many types of research, including instrument development and validation studies, experimental designs, program evaluations, institutional research and assessments, and student and other type surveys (Snow, 2012).

QRS has many advanced features that make it more useful than other browser-based survey platforms, including the following (Snow, 2012):

- Easy survey design with point-and-click editing
- A comprehensive list of question types with complex skip patterns and branching
- The capability to send personalized email messages and survey content to individual respondents
- Randomization of question order or response categories
- Authentication for linkage to other databases or preventing "ballot-box stuffing"
- The capability for respondents to stop in mid-survey and resume later where they left off
- The online generation and export of reports, graphics, PowerPoint slides, and cross-tabulations of survey results
- Simple data download to spreadsheet, SPSS, or other file formats

Data collected through QRS are stored on Qualtrics's servers unless/until downloaded by the researcher. MGH initiated its first annual contract with Qualtrics in 2010. Since January 1, 2012, 31 MGH researchers in Patient Care Services have conducted 233 new surveys using QRS and collected data on 15,745 respondents. At MGH, using QRS makes it easy to capture real-time data that is used to inform data-driven healthcare decisions.

REDCap

MGH also uses the Research Electronic Data Capture (REDCap), developed through Vanderbilt University Institute for Clinical and Translational Research in 2004 (Harris et al., 2008). REDCap is a freely available, secure, flexible, and HIPAA-compliant web-based application used for a various types of research, including clinical trials and other healthcare studies. REDCap provides easy data manipulation; audit trails for reporting, monitoring, and querying patient records; and an automated export mechanism to common statistical packages, including R/S-Plus, SAS, SPSS, and Stata. Additionally, REDCap has capabilities for designing and handling online surveys. REDCap is currently supported by the REDCap Consortium, composed of active institutional partners from research groups in healthcare agencies and other institutions worldwide. According to the consortium's website, REDCap is now available in (addition to English) Chinese, French, German, and Portuguese, with other language translations anticipated in the near future (REDCap Consortium, 2014). You can find a full description of REDCap and its available resources for users at the REDCap Consortium website (http://project-redcap.org).

Other Instruments Modeled After the PPM, PPE, or RPPE

Several instruments have been modeled after the development of the RPPE scale, including the following:

- Chinese Professional Practice Environment (CPPE) scale for Taiwanese nurses
- 2011 Staff Perceptions of the CPPE surveys
- Leadership Influence over Professional Practice Environments Scale (LIPPES)
- Australian validation of the PPE scale
- Patient Care Associates—Work Environment Scale (PCA-WES)
- Staff Perceptions of the Disruptive Patient Behavior (SPDPB) scale

The CPPE Scale for Taiwanese Nurses

Since 2008, several instruments have been developed and used to evaluate different aspects of the PPE using the original PPE scale or the RPPE scale as the basis for the development of a scale. In 2008, Chang (2009) developed a Chinese version of the original PPE, called the Chinese Professional Practice Environment (CPPE) scale, for use with Taiwanese nurses because there were no culturally sensitive instruments available to evaluate Taiwanese nurses' practice environments.

After translation of the PPE scale from English to Chinese (CPPE), 10 Taiwanese nurse experts evaluated the CPPE for semantic and content equivalence. They recommended that another element, Professional Development, be added to the scale so as to improve the CPPE's comprehensiveness and cultural sensitivity. The CPPE's content equivalence was supported by satisfactory content validity indices. Chang developed and content-validated 27 more items and added them to the CPPE, increasing its length to 66 items.

Chang then administered the CPPE to 977 Taiwanese nurses working in acute care settings. The Cronbach's alpha internal consistency reliability for the 66-item scale was 0.95. Examination of the item-total correlation of the measure revealed that two items were redundant of other, more conceptually clear items; therefore, they were dropped from the CPPE. After computing various orthogonal and oblique rotations of PCAs and factor analyses on the now 64-item CPPE, the PCA with Varimax rotation and Kaiser normalization producing an 11-component solution was judged most parsimonious and interpretable. This PCA-derived CPPE was formed by 58 of the 64 items with component loadings above the 0.30 cutoff.

The Cronbach's alpha internal consistency was 0.95 for the total 58-item CPPE and ranged from 0.71 to 0.87 for the subscales. The psychometric structure of the 58-item CPPE was different from the original PPE, which was not unexpected given the additional number of items (n = 27) added to the scale to make it more comprehensive and culturally sensitive to the Taiwanese nurses. For an in-depth discussion of the development and psychometric evaluation with accompanying tables, see Chang's dissertation (Chang, 2009). The dissertation also contains a copy of the Taiwanese version of the 66-item CPPE in Appendix N.

2011 Staff Perceptions of the CPPE Survey

In 2011, the English version of the SPPPE survey was back-translated into Mandarin Chinese (CSPPPE) with no editing for comprehensiveness or cultural sensitivity. In September 2011, the CSPPPE was then administered to a sample of 941 nurses, from 10 Chinese hospitals, who provided direct care to patients. Completed surveys were sent to research staff in the MGH Yvonne L. Munn Center for Nursing Research (Munn Center), where they were manually entered into SPSS, version 19.0. Once data entry was completed, data analysis was undertaken by a senior nurse scientist in the Munn Center. Note that no psychometric evaluation of the Mandarin Chinese version of the RPPE contained in the CSPPPE has been done yet (Duffy, Ives Erickson, Ditomassi, & Jones, 2013).

Almost all CSPPPE respondents were female (99%) and married (55%), ranging in age from 21 to 67 years, with an average age of 30 years. Their highest educational level was mostly at the diploma level (82%), with 17% having bachelor degrees and less than 1% having master or doctoral degrees. Almost all Chinese nurses worked full time (99%) on wards (55%) or in intensive care units (16%), operating rooms (8%), emergency departments (6%), or other settings (15%). Chinese respondents had spent an average of 1 year in nursing and worked in their institution 9 years and on their current unit an average of 4.5 years (Duffy et al., 2013).

The Cronbach's alpha internal consistency reliability scores for the total Mandarin Chinese RPPE score was 0.95, which indicated a very high Cronbach's alpha reliability coefficient. However, subscale scores ranged from 0.21 to 0.91, indicating that only 5 of the 8 RPPE subscales were reliable. The Communication About Patients, Teamwork, and Staff Relations with Physicians subscales exhibited internal consistency reliability coefficients that were below the 0.70 cutoff. These low coefficients could be due, in part, to the small number of items comprising each subscale as well as the fact that the Mandarin Chinese RPPE may not have been as culturally sensitive to the Chinese nurse population in these 10 hospitals.

When the Chinese RPPE subscale and work satisfaction means and standard deviations were compared to the 2011 MGH RNs' RPPE results, scores for both groups were quite similar:

- Chinese nurses and MGH nurses scored the same on the RPPE Autonomy and Leadership subscale, and Chinese RNs had slightly higher scores on the Teamwork and Handling Disagreement and Conflict subscales.

- Chinese nurses' scores were somewhat lower on the Staff Relations with Physicians, Control over Practice, Communication About Patients, Internal Work Motivation, and Cultural Sensitivity RPPE subscales than MGH nurses' scores.

- Chinese nurses' work satisfaction scores were also slightly lower than their MGH counterparts.

Note that both Chinese and MGH nurses' scores on all scales were relatively high, with all scores falling above the mean and median for that score (Duffy et al., 2013).

Leadership Influence over Professional Practice Environments Scale

The Leadership Influence over Professional Practice Environments Scale (LIPPES) was developed from a synthesis of concepts derived from the Adams Influence Model (Adams, 2008; 2009) and the RPPE scale findings (Ives Erickson at al., 2009). The original LIPPES consisted of 95 items measuring 6 components (Adams, Nikolaev, Ives Erickson, Ditomassi, & Jones, 2013):

- Authority

- Communication traits

- Knowledge-based competence

- Status

- Time and timing

- Influence and power

The items were measured on a 5-point scale with 1 = not applicable, 2 = never, 3 = sometimes, 4 = often, and 5 = always. The LIPPES was reviewed by content experts for uniformity in clarity, comprehension, and content validity. Only minor changes were made to item text (Adams et al., 2013).

Following institutional review approval, the paper version of the LIPPES was distributed at the 2010 Institute for Nursing Healthcare Leadership (INHL) conference in Boston. Attendees were exclusively nurse executives, managers, and leaders (Adams et al., 2013). In addition, the electronic version of the LIPPES was emailed to two large nursing administration organizations' listservs. Of the 289 respondents to the LIPPES, 52 returned paper copies, and 237 completed the electronic survey. No participant filled out both a paper and an electronic LIPPES survey. Because many respondents did not complete all LIPPES items, 139 cases were dropped from psychometric analyses, resulting in a sample size of 150 respondents.

Initially, the 95-item LIPPES was reduced to 59 items because of low component loadings below the 0.40 cutoff and through parceling (Little, Cunningham, Shahar, & Wideman, 2002), a measurement practice that is used most commonly in multivariate approaches to psychometrics, particularly for use with latent-variable analysis techniques (e.g., exploratory factor analysis, structural equation modeling). A parcel is defined as an aggregate-level indicator comprising the sum (or average) of two or more items, responses, or behaviors that are combined (Little et al., 2002). The internal consistency Cronbach's alpha coefficient for the now 59-item LIPPES was 0.97.

PCA with Varimax rotation and Kaiser normalization specifying a six-component structure was next calculated on the 59-item LIPPES. All items loaded above the 0.40 loading cutoff, confirming the six-component structure but not the hypothesized theoretical structure of the scale and accounting for 64% of explained variance. Closer examination of the actual PCA component structure produced two of the six hypothesized components: Authority and Status. The other four components, although different from the original hypothesized structure, made conceptual sense and could be named and interpreted as related to leadership influence and positive practice environments (Adams et al., 2013). They were named:

- Collegial Administrative Approach

- Internal Strategy and Resolve

- Access to Resources

- Leadership Expectations of Staff

Cronbach's alpha internal consistency reliability coefficients ranged from 0.89 to 0.94 on the six LIPPES subscales. So, the 59-item LIPPES scale was judged reliable and factorially valid for use in subsequent research studies. A multisite study is currently underway to continue to elevate the psychometric properties of the LIPPES scale. (Adams et al., 2013).

Australian Validation of the PPE Scale

A psychometric evaluation of the original PPE was undertaken in a sample of general practice nurses in Australia (Halcomb, Davidson, Caldwell, Salamonson, & Rolley, 2010). After editing the PPE slightly to make it appropriate for the Australian general practice setting, Halcomb and colleagues administered the adapted PPE online to all general practice nurse recipients (N = 1,123) of scholarships received through the Australian Practice Nurses Association (Halcomb et al., 2010). A sample of 342 respondents with complete data on the PPE was used for the psychometric evaluation.

The component structure of the 38-item online PPE was examined using principal components analysis with Varimax rotation and Kaiser normalization. An eight-component solution accounted for 71.6% of the variance. Low component loadings < 0.30 cutoff or cross-component loadings were detected in eight items. These items were dropped from the PPE, making it a 30-item scale.

The Cronbach's alpha internal consistency reliability coefficients for the eight PPE subscales ranged from 0.71 to 0.89 for the subscales, with 0.94 for the total score. A comparison of Cronbach's alpha values demonstrated little change in the deletion of eight items from four of the eight component subscales. Halcomb and colleagues concluded that the 30-item version of the PPE was reliable and valid for evaluating the PPE of nurses working in Australian general practice.

Patient Care Associates—Work Environment Scale

Patient care associates are very valuable and integral members of the healthcare team providing care at the bedside to patients and their families. Although professional staff caregivers at MGH were evaluated regularly using the MGH SPPPE survey, patient care associates were not included. In late 2009, MGH nursing leadership decided to undertake the first Patient Care Associates' Perceptions of the Work Environment study to provide leadership with timely feedback about patient care associates' work experience. The survey was designed to assess patient care associates' primary work environment (using the Patient Care Associate-Work Environment Scale [PCA-WES] designed for this purpose), their overall work satisfaction, and several demographic and work characteristics (Ives Erickson, Duffy, & Jones, 2015).

The PCA-WES was developed by MGH nurse scientists in the Munn Center. Initially, it was a 60-item, multidimensional measure of five components of the patient care associates' work environment:

- **Staff Attitude Toward the Patient Care Associate Role (17 items):** The patient care associates' report of the general outlook of the staff with whom they work regarding their performance

- **Patient Care Associates' Attitude Toward Work (13 items):** Their general outlook about their work, including what motivates them in their work and what they, as PCAs, contribute to patients and their families

- **Patient Care Associates' Communication with Nursing Manager/Leader (10 items):** The degree to which patient care information was relayed promptly to the people who need to be informed through open channels of discourse (Shortell et al., 1991)

- **Patient Care Associates' Teamwork (10 items):** A conscious activity designed to achieve unity of effort in the pursuit of shared objectives (Zimmerman et al., 1993)

- **Patient Care Associates' Respect for Patients and Their Families (10 items):** A set of attitudes and practices/policies that accepts others as they are

When the Patient Care Associate-Work Environment Scale test pool was completed, a panel of five MGH patient care associates reviewed the items for content validity by determining the extent to which each item represented the conceptual category it was designed to measure. Their review of the items for readability, clarity, and meaning resulted in minor wording changes to several items; all items were retained. Each item was placed on a four-point Likert scale of N (never), S (sometimes), O (often), and A (always). A brief set of instructions was developed to guide patient care associate test-takers by asking them to think about the unit on which they usually work and to circle the letter on the four-point response scale that best indicated the degree to which the statement applied.

Munn Center nurse scientists conducted the PCA-WES study in late spring, 2009. After receiving approval from the MGH Institutional Review Board, all MGH patient care associates (N = 463) were invited to participate in the study. Survey packets containing a letter of invitation to participate in the study, the PCA-WES survey, and a stamped and addressed return envelope were mailed to patient care associate' home addresses. Patient care associates were assured that participation in the study was voluntary and that all responses would be kept anonymous. They were also asked whether they wished any written comment they made on the survey to be shared with others. Patient care associates' return of completed surveys served as their consent to participate in the study. A total of 229 MGH patient care associates returned such surveys.

In 2011, nursing leadership at New York University Langone Medical Center (NYULMC) were asked to participate in the PCA-WES study and agreed to do so. Nurse scientists in the MGH Munn Center conducted another survey in the late spring 2011 after approval was secured from the Institutional Review Board. Of the 420 eligible to participate at NYULMC, 205 returned completed surveys. Their return of these surveys indicated their consent to participate in the study.

Data from the MGH (n = 229) and NYULMC (n = 205) surveys were combined to produce a sample size of 434 patient care associates. Of this number, 44 respondents had missing data on the PCA-WES and were dropped from the sample. This sample of 390 patient care associates from the two institutions with no missing data on the 60 items was used to undertake a psychometric evaluation of the PCA-WES. This evaluation included:

- Internal consistency reliability using Cronbach's alpha

- Principal components analysis with Varimax rotation and Kaiser normalization

- Internal consistency reliability of resulting components using Cronbach's alpha

The evaluation went as follows:

1. Item-total correlations were computed for the 60-item PCA-WES.

   The Cronbach's alpha was 0.95 for the total scale, with 24 items having item-total correlations below the 0.30 cutoff. These items were dropped, and 36 PCA-WES items with item-total correlations > 0.30 were subjected to principal components analysis (PCA).

2. The PCA was followed by Varimax rotation, and Kaiser normalization was performed on the sample.

   Initially, there were seven components with eigenvalues > 1, explaining 64.1% of variance. An examination of this rotated solution was uninterpretable.

3. The scree test was inspected, indicating a five-component solution.

4. Because the PCA-WES was designed to measure five dimensions, a PCA specifying five components was calculated and examined.

   After inspection of the PCA rotated component matrix, the researchers judged the 5-component solution to be both parsimonious and interpretable.

All but 1 of the 36 items loaded greater than the 0.30 loading cutoff on one of the five components. There were very few substantial side loadings. The five PCA-derived scales accounted for a total of 57.2% of initially extracted common variance:

- Component 1, labeled Staff Attitude Toward the Patient Care Associate Role (12 items), accounted for 21.0% of variance.

- Component 2, called Patient Care Associates' Attitude Toward Work (13 items), explained an additional 14.9% of variance.

- Component 3, called Patient Care Associates' Communication with Nursing Manager/Leader (5 items), added 9.2% of variance.

- Component 4, named Patient Care Associates' Teamwork (3 items), explained an additional 6.6% of variance.

- Component 5, labeled Patient Care Associates' Respect for Patients and Their Families (2 items), explained an additional 5.5% of variance.

These five components accounted for a total of 57.2% of explained variance. Cronbach's alpha internal consistency reliabilities for each of the five PCA-WES components ranged from 0.84 to 0.93. So, the now 35-item PCA-WES measuring five major components of patient care associates' work environment was judged sufficiently reliable and valid for use as independent measures in subsequent research (Ives Erickson, Duffy, & Jones, 2015).

Staff Perceptions of the Disruptive Patient Behavior Scale

Disruptive patient behavior (DPB), including physical/verbal aggression toward nurses, has a major impact on work safety within today's hospitals. The DPB rate, predominantly with nurses, has increased recently, a finding locally confirmed by a doubling in DPB reporting within MGH (Lipkis-Orlando, Carroll, Duffy, Weiss, & Jones, 2014). This increase raised concerns about the MGH staff's recognition of DPB risk factors, their preparedness to manage DPB, their knowledge and use of resources, and their perceptions of leadership support.

After undertaking a search of extant literature, Lipkis-Orlando and colleagues (2014) concluded that despite the importance of the issue, no standardized approach to benchmarking the DPB experience was available to guide the development of knowledge-based interventions to deal with DPB in the clinical practice setting. To this end, the mixed-methods study was undertaken to develop an instrument that would measure MGH clinical staffs' knowledge about DPB and how best to handle this complex occurrence.

Following Institutional Review Board approval, phase one of the study took place:

1. Four open-ended qualitative questions focused on the experience, attitudes, and management of DPB, in addition to post-event responses, were developed as an online survey.

2. The open-ended survey was emailed to MGH clinical and nonclinical staff on inpatient units, the emergency department, and ambulatory care practices.

   MGH survey respondents (N = 770), 70% of which were nurses, completed the open-ended survey.

3. The responses were analyzed using content analysis and theme identification (Lipkis-Orlando et al., 2014).

4. Each theme was defined, followed by a selection of representative quotes that actualized the respective theme.

   The major DPB themes identified were as follows (Lipkis-Orlando et al., 2014):

   - Preventive approaches, including better management of neuropsychiatric conditions
   - Ready access to training and expertise that includes security staff and psychiatric consultation
   - The value of post-event follow-up for staff support
   - Clinical guidelines development

5. The themes were reviewed by a panel of experts who concluded that the content and thematic analyses showed good overall fit with extant literature.

6. A prototype 66-item instrument was generated and reviewed by the expert panel for content validity, legibility, readability, and comprehensibility (Lipkis-Orlando et al., 2014).

Then in phase two of the study:

1. The 66-item scale, called the Staff Perceptions of the Disruptive Patient Behavior (SPDPB) scale, was converted to an online survey using Qualtrics, a web-based platform discussed previously (Snow, 2012).

2. In March 2013, all 2,938 MGH direct care nurses received an invitation letter to fill out the SPDPB scale on the Qualtrics website.

   Of this number, 558 MGH nurses completed the 66-item online SPDPB scale. The Cronbach's alpha internal consistency reliability coefficient for the SPDPB scale was 0.95.

3. PCA followed by Varimax rotation and Kaiser normalization was performed on the sample (N = 558), resulting in 11 components with eigenvalues > 1, explaining 63.3% of variance.

4. The scree test was inspected, indicating a six-component solution.

5. A PCA specifying six components was calculated and examined.

After inspection of the PCA rotated component matrix, the researchers judged this six-component solution to be the most parsimonious and interpretable. All but 1 of the 66 items loaded greater than the 0.30 component loading cutoff on one of the six components. If an item had a significant side loading greater than 0.30 on more than one component, the highest number was considered as the defining loading:

- Component 1, labeled Leadership Support for Dealing with Disruptive Behavior (16 items), accounted for 13.0% of variance.

- Component 2, called Staff Actions Related to Disruptive Behavior (14 items), explained an additional 12.7% of variance.

- Component 3, called Overall Staff Preparation and Attitude Toward Disruptive Behavior (15 items), added 9.5% of variance.

- Component 4, named Staff Experience of Disruptive Behavior (10 items), explained an additional 8.7% of variance.

- Component 5, labeled Staff Skills in Handling Disruptive Behavior (6 items), explained an additional 5.8% of variance.

- Component 6, called Security Personnel Response to Disruptive Behavior (4 items), added 4.4% of explained variance.

These six components accounted for a total of 54.1% of explained variance. The Cronbach's alpha internal consistency reliability coefficients for the six sub-scales ranged from 0.78 to 0.93. So, the now 65-item SPDPB scale measuring six major components of health providers' experience of DPB when giving direct care to patients was judged sufficiently reliable and valid for use in subsequent research (Lipkis-Orlando et al., 2014).

Publications Springing from the PPM/PPE/RPPE

In addition to the research reported in this chapter, a number of other reports by MGH and other nurse researchers have been published in the past several years. The following sections list them by year of publication, with no attempt to summarize these reports. You are encouraged to review the published reports for more complete information.

2014 Publications

Carroll, D. (2014). The effects of intensive care unit environments on nurse perception of family presence during resuscitation and invasive procedures. *Dimensions of Critical Care Nursing 33*(1), 34–39.

Papastavrou, E., Efstathiou, G., Lemonidou, C., Kalafati, M., Katajisto, J., & Suhonen, R. (2014). Cypriot and Greek nurses perceptions of the professional practice environment. *International Nursing Review, 6*(2), 171–178.

Suhonen, R., Stolt, M., Gustafsson, M., Katajisto, J., & Charalambous, A. (2014). The associations among the ethical climate, the professional practice environment and individualized care in care settings for older people. *Journal of Advanced Nursing, 70*(6), 1356–68.

2013 Publications

Cronin, J., Keeley, A., & Blakeney, B. (2013). Transforming a unit: The impact of care innovation and transformation promoting change and empowering new leaders. *American Organization of Nurse Executives*, September, 4-5.

Dykes, P., Carroll, D., Hurley, A., Benoit, A., Chang, F., Pozzar, R., & Caligtan, C. (2013). Building and testing a patient-centric electronic bedside communication center. *Journal of Gerontological Nursing, 39*(1), 15–19.

Edwards, E., Despotopulos, L., & Carroll, D. (2013). Interventions to support family presence in the cardiac intensive care unit. *Clinical Nurse Specialist, 27*(5), 2379–244.

Hill, R., Vorderstrasse, A., Turner, B., Pereira, K., & Thompson, J. (2013). Screening for depression in patients with diabetes: Addressing the challenge. *The Journal for Nurse Practitioners, 9*(4), 208–213.

Ives Erickson, J. (2013). Reflections on leadership talent: A void or an opportunity? *Nursing Administration Quarterly, 37*(1), 44–51.

Ives Erickson, J., Jones, D., & Ditomassi, M. (2013). *Fostering nurse-led care: professional practice for the bedside leader from massachusetts general hospital.* Indianapolis IN: Sigma Theta Tau International.

Larkin, M., Staten, M., Wexler, D., & Lachin, J. (2013). GRADE study research group: Rationale and design of the glycemia reduction approaches in diabetes: A comparative effectiveness study. *Diabetes Care, 10*(Supplement 1), 43–55.

Mulready-Shick, J., Flanagan, K., Banister, G., Mylott, L., & Curtin, L. (2013). Evaluating dedicated education units for clinical education quality. *Journal of Nursing Education, 52*(11), 606–614.

Perry, D. (2013). Transcendental method for research with human subjects: A transformational phenomenology for the human sciences. *Field Methods, 36*(3), 171–185.

Richards, D., Larkin, M., Javier, E., Casey, T., & Grey, M. (2013). Learning needs of youth with type 2 diabetes. *The Diabetes Educator Journal, 39*(3), 314–319.

2012 Publications

Barba, K., & Mahan Butt, T. (2012). *Nursing care of the hospitalized older patient.* Wiley-Blackwell.

Grace, P., & Robinson, E. (2013). Nursing's moral imperative. In J. Ives Erickson, M. Ditomassi, & D. Jones (Eds.), *Fostering Nurse-Led Care: Professional Practice for the Bedside Leader* (pp. 123–152). Indianapolis, IN: Sigma Theta Tau International.

Ives Erickson, J., Ditomassi, M., & Adams, J. (2012). Developing the leadership skill set for the executive nurse leader. In S. Ahmed, L. Andrist, S. Davis, S., & V. Fuller (Eds.), *DNP Education, Practice, and Policy: Redesigning Advanced Practice Roles for the 21st Century* (pp. 137–148). Springer Publishing Company.

Logan, J. (1994). *The relationship of decentralized organizational structure to perceived aspects of the professional nursing practice environment.* University of Ottawa (Canada), PhD dissertation.

Parker, K., & Smith, C. (2012). Assessment and planning for a dedicated education unit. *Journal for Nurses in Staff Development, 28*(3), E1–8.

2011 and Earlier Publications

Adams, J. M. (2011). Influencing the future of nursing. *JONA, 41*(10), 394–396.

Carroll, D., Dykes, P., & Hurley, A. (2010). Patients' perspectives of falling while in an acute care hospital and suggestions for prevention. *Applied Nursing Research, 23*(4), 238–241.

Clarke, P., & Jones, D. (2011). Expanding consciousness in nursing education and practice. *Nursing Science Quarterly, 24*(3), 223–226.

Jones, D., Duffy, M., & Flanagan, J. (2011). Randomized clinical trial testing the efficacy of a nurse-coached intervention in arthroscopy patients. *Nursing Research, 60*(2), 92–99.

Lee, S., & Coakley, E. (2011). Geropalliative care: A concept synthesis. *Journal of Hospice & Palliative Care Nursing, 13*(4), 242–248

Pai, H., Lee, S., & Chang T. (2011). A confirmatory factor analysis of the Clinical Nursing Practice Environment Scale with hospital registered nurses in Taiwan. *Journal of Clinical Nursing, 20,* (15–16) 2344–2354.

Wolf, L. (2011). *Testing and refining an integrated ethically-driven environmental model of clinical decision-making in emergency settings.* Boston College, PhD dissertation.

Charalambous A., Katajisto J., Välimäki, M., Leino-Kilpi, H., & Suhonen, R. (2010). Individualized care and the professional practice environment: Nurses' perceptions. *International Nursing Review, 57*(4), 500–507.

Adams, J. M., Ives Erickson, J., Jones, D. A., & Paulo, L. (2009). An evidence based structure for transformative nurse executive practice: The model of the interrelationship of leadership, environments & outcomes for nurse executives (MILE ONE). *Nursing Administration Quarterly, 33*(4), 280–287.

Breckenridge-Sproat, S. (2009). *Unit-level staffing, workload, and adverse events in army acute care hospitals: 2003–2006.* University of Maryland, Baltimore, PhD dissertation.

Carroll, D. L., & Gonzalez, C. E. (2009). Visiting preferences of cardiovascular patients. *Progress in Cardiovascular Nursing, 24*(4), 149–154.

Dykes, P. C., Carroll, D. L., Hurley, A., Lipsitz, S., Benoit, A., Chang, F., Meltzer, S., Tsurikova, R., Zuyov, L. & Middleton, B. (2010). Fall prevention in acute care hospitals: A randomized trial. *JAMA, 304*(17), 1912–1918.

Hawes, K. (2009). *Nurse job stress, burnout, practice environment, and maternal satisfaction in the neonatal intensive care unit.* University of Rhode Island, PhD dissertation.

Ives Erickson, J., Duffy, M., Ditomassi, M., & Jones, D. (2009). Psychometric evaluation of the revised professional practice environment (RPPE). *JONA, 39*(5), 1–8.

Lee, S., Coakley, E., Dahlin, C., & Ford-Carleton, P. (2009). An evidence-based nurse residency program in geropalliative care. *Journal of Continuing Education in Nursing, 40*(12), 536–542.

Logan, J. (1994). *The relationship of decentralized organizational structure to perceived aspects of professional nursing practice environment.* University of Ottawa (Canada), PhD dissertation.

Summary

The findings cited in this chapter show that the Australian-adapted, English, and Chinese versions of the multidimensional PPE and RPPE are psychometrically sound measures of various components of the professional practice environment in both acute and general practice settings. These scales also demonstrate substantive coherence and application at both the individual and one or more organizational levels of analysis. Three newer instruments, the LIPPES, PCA-WES, and SPDPB scales have demonstrated psychometric adequacy. In addition, all measures are linked to a professional practice model that seeks to provide valuable information describing effective PPEs. Such information is useful in helping nursing leadership design, improve, and evaluate the various components of an individual unit or department practice setting, thus giving them important information about whether changes have made a difference in practice. Finally, the number of research projects, grant proposals, funded projects, and related publications continues to grow at the MGH, an organization committed to nursing research and interdisciplinary research collaborations that foster high-quality, safe, efficient, patient-family centric care.

References

Adams, J. (2008). *Validation of the Adams Influence Model (AIM)*. Boston College: PhD dissertation.

Adams. J. (2009). *The Adams Influence Model (AIM): Understanding the Factors, Attributes and Process of Achieving Influence*. Saarbruken, Germany: VDM Verlag.

Adams, J., Nikolaev, N., Ives Erickson, J., Ditomassi, M., & Jones D. (2013). Identification of the psychometric properties of the leadership influence over professional practice environments scale. *Journal of Nursing Administration, 43*(5), 258–265.

Aiken, L., Havens, D., & Sloan, D. (2000). The Magnet Nursing Services Recognition Program: A comparison or two groups of Magnet® hospitals. *American Journal of Nursing, 100*(3), 26–36.

Aiken, L., Sochalski, J., & Lake, E. (1997). Studying outcomes of organizational change in health services. *Medical Care, 35*(11 Supplement), N58-N518.

Barrett E.A.M (1989). A nursing theory of power for nursing practice; Derivation from Rogers paradigm. In J. Riehl (Ed.) *Conceptual models for nursing practice* (3rd Ed.). (pp 207-217). Norwalk, CT; Appleton & Lange

Barrett E.A.M (1990a). A measure of power as knowing participation in change. In O. Strickland & C. Waltz (Eds.). *The measurement of nursing outcomes: Measuring client self-care and coping skills* (Vol. 4) (pp. 159-180). New York; Springer

Blakeney, B., Carleton, P., McCarthy, C., & Coakley, E. (2009). Unlocking the power of innovation. *OJIN: The Online Journal of Issues in Nursing*. Retrieved from http://www.nursingworld.org/MainMenuCategories/ANAMarketplace/ANAPeriodicals/OJIN/TableofContents/Vol142009/No2May09/Innovation.html

Brayfield, A.H., & Rothe, H.F. An index of job satisfaction. *Journal of Applied Psychology, 35(5),* 307-311

Caroselli, C. & Barrett, E.A.M. (1998b). A review of the power as knowing participation in change literature. *Nursing Science Quarterly, 11* 9-16

Chang, C. (2009). Development and Evaluation of Psychometric Properties of the Chinese Version of the Professional Practice Environment Scale in Taiwan (Unpublished doctoral dissertation). Boston College.

Cudeck, R., & Brown, M. (1983). Cross-validation of covariance structures. *Multivariate Behavioral Research, 18,* 147–167.

Duffy, M., Ives Erickson J., Ditomassi, M., & Jones, D. (2013). Measuring the hospital work environment with the professional practice environment scale: Development, validation and revision. In J. Ives Erickson, M. Ditomassi, & D. Jones (Eds.), *Fostering Nurse-Led Care: Professional Practice for the Bedside Leader* (275–305). Indianapolis, IN: Sigma Theta Tau International.

EdTech Times Staff. (2014). University-wide adoption of qualtrics research suite grows by 40 percent. Retrieved from: http://edtechtimes.com/2014/04/23/university-wide-qualtrics-grows-40-percent/

Fry, S., & Duffy, M. (2001). Development & psychometric evaluation of the ethical issues scale. *Journal of Nursing Scholarship, 33*(3), 273–277.

Hackman, J., & Oldham, G. (1976). Motivation through the design of work: Test of a theory. *Organizational Behavior and Human Performance, 16*(2), 250–279.

Hackman, J., & Oldham, G. (1980). *Work re-design*. Reading, MA: Addison-Wesley.

Halcomb, E., Davidson, P., Caldwell, B., Salamonson, Y., & Rolley, J. (2010, 2nd Quarter). Validation of the professional practice environment scale in Australian general practice. *Journal of Nursing Scholarship, 42*(2), 207–213.

Harris, P., Thielke, R., Taylor, J., Payne, N., Gonzalez, J., & Conde, J. (2008). Research Electronic Data Capture (REDCap): A metadata-driven methodology and workflow process for providing translational research informatics support. *Journal of Biomedical Informatics, 42*(2), 377–381.

Institute of Medicine (IOM). (2001). *Crossing the quality chasm: A new health system for the 21st century*. Washington, DC: National Academies Press.

Ives Erickson, J. (2000, July 20). Keeping in touch with staff perceptions of the professional practice environment. *Caring Headlines*, 2.

Ives Erickson, J. (2012). 200 years of nursing—A chief nurse's reflections on practice, theory, policy, education and research. *Journal of Nursing Administration, 42*(1), 9–11.

Ives Erickson, J., & Ditomassi, M. (2011). Professional practice model: Strategies for translating models into practice. *Nursing Clinics of North America 46* (35–44). Elsevier.

Ives Erickson, J., Duffy, M., Ditomassi, M., & Jones, D. (2009). Psychometric evaluation of the revised professional practice environment scale. *Journal of Nursing Administration, 39*(5), 236–243.

Ives Erickson, J., Duffy, M., Gibbons, M., Fitzmaurice, J., & Ditomassi, M. (2004). Development and psychometric evaluation of the professional practice environment scale. *Journal of Nursing Scholarship, 36*(3), 279–285.

Ives Erickson, J., Duffy, M., & Jones, D. (2015). Development and psychometric evaluation of the patient care associates work environment scale. *Journal of Nursing Administration, 45*(3), 139–144.

Koloroutis, M., (Ed.). (2004). *Relationship-based care: A model for transforming practice*. Minneapolis, MN: Creative Health Care Management.

Lake, E. (2002). Development of the practice environment scale of the nursing work index. *Research in Nursing & Health, 25*, 176–188.

Lipkis-Orlando, R., Carroll, D., Duffy, M., Weiss, A., & Jones, D. (2014). Psychometric evaluation of the staff perception of the disruptive patient behavior scale. Unpublished manuscript.

Little, T., Cunningham, W., Shahar, G., & Widaman, K. (2002). To parcel or not to parcel: Exploring the question, weighing the merits. *Structural Equation Modeling, 9*(2), 151–173.

McClure, M., Poulin, M., Sovie, M., & Wandelt, M. (1983). *Magnet® Hospitals: Attraction and Retention of Professional Nurses*. (ANA Publication G-160), Washington, DC: American Academy of Nursing.

Nunnally, J., & Bernstein, L. (1994). *Psychometric theory* (3rd ed.). New York: McGraw-Hill.

REDCap Consortium (2014). *REDCap: Research Electronic Data Capture*. Retrieved from http://project-redcap.org/

Relationship-based care. (n.d.) Retrieved from http://chcm.com/relationship-based-care/

Sackett, D., Straus S., Richardson, W., Rosenberg, W., & Haynes, R. (2000). *Evidence-based medicine: How to practice and teach EBM*. Edinburgh: Churchill Livingstone.

Sherman, R., & Pross, E. (2010, January 31). Growing future nurse leaders to build and sustain healthy work environments at the unit level. *OJIN: The Online Journal of Issues in Nursing 15*(1), Manuscript 1.

Shortell, S., Rousseau, D., Gillies, R., Devers, K., & Simons, T. (1991). Organizational assessment in intensive care units (ICUs): Construct development, reliability and validity of the ICU nurse-physician questionnaire. *Medical Care, 29*, 709–723.

Snow, J. (2012). *Qualtrics survey software: Handbook for research professionals.* Provo, UT: Qualtrics Labs Inc.

Zimmerman, J., Shortell, S., Rousseau, D., Duffy, J., Gillies, R., Knaus, W., Devers, K., Wagner, D., & Draper, E. (1993). Improving intensive care: Observations based on organizational case studies in nine intensive care units. *Critical Care Medicine, 21*(10), 1443–1551.

Chapter 9

The Magnet Recognition Program® Journey: An Engine for Research and Evidence-Based Practice

–Marianne Ditomassi, DNP, MBA, RN

The Magnet Recognition Program® has been a strong force in promoting hospital-based nursing research since its inception. Wilson, Kelly, Reifsnider, Pipe, and Brumfield (2013) note that nursing research provides the foundation for evidence-based nursing practice (EBP). Both research generation and the integration of evidence into practice are hallmarks of a Magnet®-recognized organization (Drenkard, 2013).

Grounded in Research

The Magnet Recognition Program® is grounded in research. Linda H. Aiken, PhD, RN, FAAN, FRCN in her presidential address to the American Academy of Nursing in September 1980, presented the following challenge (Aiken, 1981, p. 325; McClure, Poulin, Sovie, & Wandelt, 1983, p. 1; McClure & Hinshaw, 2002, p. 1):

> *"Despite an aggregate national supply of nurses that is larger than ever before, over 80 percent of America's hospitals do not have adequate*

nursing staffs. There are currently some 100,000 vacancies in hospital nursing positions and this has had a crippling effect on the day-to-day operations of many hospitals."

In response to this challenge, the American Academy of Nursing in 1981 authorized a study to answer two main questions:

- What are the important variables in the hospital organization and its nursing service that create a magnetism that attracts and retains professional nurses on its staff?

- What particular combination of variable produces model(s) of hospital nursing practice in which nurses receive professional and personal satisfaction to the degree that recruitment and retention of qualified staff are achieved? (McClure et al., 1983, p. 2-3; McClure & Hinshaw, 2002, p .2).

Out of more than 150 hospitals nominated by fellows of the Academy for the study, the researchers eventually identified 41 that served "as 'magnets' for professional nurses—effective in attracting and retaining a staff of well-qualified nurses and are therefore consistently able to provide quality care" (McClure et al., 1983, p. 2; McClure & Hinshaw, 2002, p. 3-4)

Results of the study identified essential characteristics that needed to be present in a strong professional practice environment (PPE) that aggregate into three main categories: administration, professional practice and professional development. The 14 characteristics are referred to as the Forces of Magnetism.* Together, these drive the delivery of safe, quality care (Urden & Monarch, 2002, p. 106–107; ANCC, 2004, p. 2-3):

1. **Quality of nursing leadership:** Nursing leaders were perceived as knowledgeable, strong risk-takers who followed an articulated philosophy in the day-to-day operations of the nursing department. Nursing leaders also conveyed a strong sense of advocacy and support on behalf of the staff.

2. **Organizational structure:** Organizational structures were characterized as flat, rather than tall, and where unit-based decision-making prevailed. Nursing departments were decentralized, with strong nursing representation evident in the organizational committee structure. The nursing leader

*Forces of Magnetism is copyrighted material of the American Nurses Credentialing Center. All rights reserved. Reproduced with the permission of the American Nurses Credentialing Center.

served at the executive level of the organization, and the chief nursing officer reported to the chief executive officer.

3. **Management style:** Hospital and nursing administrators were found to use a participative management style, incorporating feedback from staff at all levels of the organization. Feedback was characterized as encouraged and valued. Nurses serving in leadership positions were visible, accessible, and committed to communicating effectively with staff.

4. **Personnel policies and programs:** Salaries and benefits were characterized as competitive. Rotating shifts were minimized, and creative and flexible staffing models were used. Personnel policies were created with staff involvement, and significant administrative and clinical promotional opportunities existed.

5. **Professional models of care:** Models of care were used that gave nurses the responsibility and authority for the provision of patient care. Nurses were accountable for their own practice and were the coordinators of care.

6. **Quality of care:** Nurses perceived that they were providing high-quality care to their patients. Providing quality care was seen as an organizational priority as well, and nurses serving in leadership positions were viewed as responsible for developing the environment in which high-quality care could be provided.

7. **Quality improvement:** Quality improvement activities were viewed as educational. Staff nurses participated in the quality improvement process and perceived the process as one that improved the quality of care delivered within the organization.

8. **Consultation and resources:** Adequate consultation and other human resources were available. Knowledgeable experts, particularly advanced practice nurses, were available and used. In addition, peer support was given within and outside the nursing division.

9. **Autonomy:** Nurses were permitted and expected to practice autonomously, consistent with professional standards. Independent judgment was expected to be exercised within the context of a multidisciplinary approach to patient care.

10. **Community and the hospital:** Hospitals that were best able to recruit and retain nurses also maintained a strong community presence. A community presence was seen in a variety of ongoing, long-term outreach programs. These outreach programs resulted in the hospital being perceived as a strong, positive, and productive corporate citizen.

11. **Nurses as teachers:** Nurses were permitted and expected to incorporate teaching in all aspects of their practice. Teaching was one activity that reportedly gave nurses a great deal of professional satisfaction.

12. **Image of nursing:** Nurses were viewed as integral to the hospital's ability to provide patient care services. The services provided by nurses were characterized as essential to other members of the healthcare team.

13. **Interdisciplinary relationships:** Interdisciplinary relationships were characterized as positive. A sense of mutual respect was exhibited among all disciplines.

14. **Professional development:** Significant emphasis was placed on orientation, in-service education, continuing education, formal education, and career development. Personal and professional growth and development were valued. In addition, opportunities for competency-based clinical advancement existed, along with the resources to maintain competency.

Magnet Recognition Program®

In the early 1990s, the board of directors of the American Nurses Association (ANA) approved a pilot project for conducting a program of evaluation based on the concepts of magnetism identified by the original Magnet® research and subsequent studies on creating a strong PPE. In addition to the 14 Forces of Magnetism that served as the framework for the Magnet Recognition Program®, other key documents were key in creating the program's foundation, including the following:

- ANA's Scope and Standards of Practice for Nurse Administrators (1995, 2004b)

- ANA Code of Ethics for Nurses (2001b), ANA Nursing's Social Policy Statement (2003)

- State Nursing Practice and Regulation Acts and Specialty Organization's Professional Standards and Guidelines (McClure & Hinshaw, 2002)

The successful pilot evolved into the Magnet Recognition Program, overseen by the ANCC, a subsidiary of the ANA. The Forces of Magnetism has served as the lens for examining the relationships that function across units and disciplines in healthcare organizations. The Magnet Recognition Program has been effective in recognizing excellence in:

- The management, philosophy, and practice of nursing services

- Adherence to national standards for improving the quality of patient care services

- Support for professional practice and continued competence of nurses

- Understanding and respecting the cultural and ethnic diversity of patients, their significant others, and healthcare providers (McClure & Hinshaw, 2002; Urden & Monarch, 2002, p. 104)

In 2007, the ANCC commissioned a statistical analysis of the final appraisal scores for applicants under the Magnet Recognition Program® Recognizing Excellence in Nursing Services Application Manual 2005 (ANCC, 2004). The project goal was to examine the relationships among the Forces of Magnetism by investigating alternative frameworks for structuring the Sources of Evidence and to inform the development of a new Magnet® Model. This new Magnet Model would provide a new perspective on the Sources of Evidence and how they interplay to create a work environment that supports excellence in nursing practice (ANCC, 2004).

As described in the Recognizing Nursing Excellence: Magnet Recognition Program® Application Manual (ANCC, 2008), through the use of a combination of factor analysis, cluster analysis, and multidimensional scaling, final Sources of Evidence scores were examined to determine how they might be organized based solely on their empirical properties. The results suggested an alternative framework for grouping the Sources of Evidence, collapsing them into fewer domains than the 14 Forces of Magnetism. The empiric model yielded from this analysis informed the conceptual development of the new Magnet® Model comprising five model components: transformational leadership; structural empowerment; exemplary professional practice; new knowledge, innovations, and improvements; and empirical outcomes (see Figure 9.1; ANCC, 2008). The following sections discuss each of the Magnet® Model components.

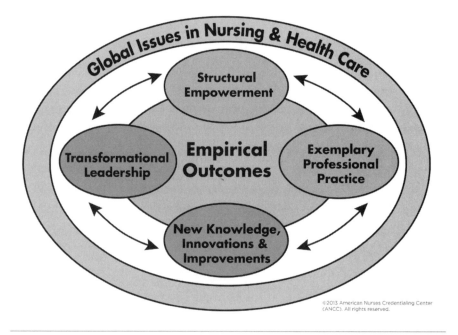

FIGURE 9.1

Magnet® Model ©2013 American Nurses Credentialing Center. All rights reserved. Reproduced with the permission of the American Nurses Credentialing Center.

Magnet® Model Components

(ANCC, www.nursecredentialing.org/magnet/programoverview/new-magnet-model)

I. Transformational Leadership

Today's healthcare environment is experiencing unprecedented, intense reformation. Unlike yesterday's leadership requirement for stabilization and growth, today's leaders must transform their organization's values, beliefs, and behaviors. It is relatively easy to lead people where they want to go; the transformational leader must lead people where they need to meet the demands of the future. This requires vision, influence, clinical knowledge, and a strong expertise relating to professional nursing practice. It also acknowledges that transformation may create turbulence and involve atypical approaches to solutions.

The organization's senior leadership team creates the vision for the future and the systems and environment necessary to achieve that vision. They must enlighten the organization as to why change is necessary and communicate each department's part in achieving that change. They must listen, challenge, influence, and affirm as the organization makes its way into the future. Gradually, this transformational way of thinking should take root in the organization and become even stronger as other leaders adapt to this way of thinking. The intent of this model component is no longer just to solve problems, fix broken systems, and empower staff, but to actually transform the organizations to meet the future. Magnet®-recognized organizations today strive for stabilization. However, healthcare reformation calls for a type of controlled destabilization that births new ideas and innovations.

II. Structural Empowerment

Solid structures and processes developed by influential leadership provide an innovative environment where strong professional practice flourishes and where the mission, vision, and values come to life to achieve the outcomes believed to be important for the organization. Further strengthening practice are the strong relationships and partnerships developed among all types of community organizations to improve patient outcomes and the health of the communities they serve. This is accomplished through the organization's strategic plan, structure, systems, policies, and programs. Staff need to be developed, directed, and empowered to find the best way to accomplish the organizational goals and achieve desired outcomes. This may be accomplished through a variety of structures and programs; one size does not fit all.

III. Exemplary Professional Practice

The true essence of a Magnet®-recognized organization stems from exemplary professional practice within nursing. This entails a comprehensive understanding of the role of nursing; the application of that role with patients, families, communities, and the interdisciplinary team; and the application of new knowledge and evidence. The goal of this component is more than the establishment of strong professional practice; it is what that professional practice can achieve.

IV. New Knowledge, Innovations, and Improvements

Strong leadership, empowered professionals, and exemplary practice are essential building blocks for Magnet®-recognized organizations, but they are not the final goals.

The ANCC states the following on its website:

> "Magnet organizations have an ethical and professional responsibility to contribute to patient care, the organization, and the profession in terms of new knowledge, innovations, and improvements. Our current systems and practices need to be redesigned and redefined if we are to be successful in the future. This component includes new models of care, application of existing evidence, new evidence, and visible contributions to the science of nursing." (www.nursecredentialing.org/magnet/ programoverview/new-magnet-model)

The Magnet® Model component of new knowledge, innovations, and improvements challenges organizations and their leadership to develop a culture encouraging inquiry, question the status quo, and focus on finding solutions to questions and problems. The Sources of Evidence for this component are organized in three elements: research, EBP, and innovation (Luzinski, 2012), which the next section discusses.

Empirical Outcomes

Magnet®-recognized organizations are in a unique position to become pioneers of the future and to demonstrate solutions to numerous problems inherent in our healthcare systems today. They may do this in a variety of ways through innovative structure and various processes, and they ought to be recognized, not penalized, for their inventiveness. In addition to strong structure and processes, they must be able to answer the question, "What difference have you made?"

Outcomes need to be categorized in terms of clinical outcomes related to nursing; workforce outcomes, patient and consumer outcomes, and organizational outcomes. When possible, outcomes data that the organization already collects should be utilized. Quantitative benchmarks should be established. These outcomes will represent the "report card" of a Magnet-recognized organization and a simple way of demonstrating excellence (www.nursecredentialing.org/magnet/programoverview/new-magnet-model).

Research and Evidence-Based Practice

Karen Drenkard (2013, p. 245) notes that Magnet®-recognized organizations promote a culture of inquiry leading to new knowledge, innovations, and improvements. The requirements for Magnet Recognition Program® evidence submission have evolved over the years. Table 9.1 lists the Sources of Evidence for research and EBP from the 2002, 2005, and 2008 Magnet Recognition Program Application Manuals. (Of note, the 2014 Magnet® Application Manual, with updated Sources of Evidence, is available for purchase from the ANCC.) Drenkard (2013) shared that requirements include completing at least one Institutional Review Board (IRB)-approved nursing research study, sharing the results, and disseminating the findings to internal and external audiences. Magnet Recognition Program requirements also include the application of EBP in the clinical setting. This can include the use of evidence-based findings to implement a practice new to the organization or to revise an existing practice to improve care.

TABLE 9.1   Magnet® Sources of Evidence: Research and Evidence-Based Practice – 2002, 2005, 2008 Application Manuals

SOURCES OF EVIDENCE: 2002	SOURCES OF EVIDENCE: 2005	SOURCES OF EVIDENCE: 2008
Criterion 13.1 Fosters the identification of areas suitable for nursing research. **Evidence:** Demonstrate that quality assessment and improvement efforts are data-based and lend themselves to the identification of areas suitable to research. It should demonstrate collaboration of the Nurse Administrator and nurses serving in leadership positions, as well as nurses who provide direct patient care with nurse researchers and researchers from other disciplines in identifying suitable research problems.	**Force 6.22** Describe how current literature, appropriate to the practice setting, is available, disseminated, and used to change administrative and clinical practices.	**NK1** Describe and demonstrate that nurses at all levels evaluate and use published research findings in their practice.

SOURCES OF EVIDENCE: 2002	SOURCES OF EVIDENCE: 2005	SOURCES OF EVIDENCE: 2008
Criterion 13.2 Supports procedures for review of proposed research studies, including protection of the rights of human subjects. **Evidence:** Provide written procedures reflecting adequate review of proposed and ongoing research studies. Involved staff must be cognizant of the need to protect human rights. Documentation must include minutes of Institutional Review Board (IRB) or equivalent; minutes of pharmacy and Therapeutics Committee (if drug studies are in place); policies and procedures for protecting the rights of human subjects; and records of training programs in the protections of human rights for staff involved in research.	**Force 6.23** Discuss the institution's policies and procedures that protect the rights of participants in research protocols. Include evidence of consistent nursing involvement in the governing body responsible for protection of human subjects in research.	**NK2** Consistent membership and involvement by at least one nurse in the governing body responsible for the protection of human subjects in research, and that a nurse votes on nursing-related protocols.

continues

TABLE 9.1 *continued*

SOURCES OF EVIDENCE: 2002	SOURCES OF EVIDENCE: 2005	SOURCES OF EVIDENCE: 2008
Criterion 13.3 Facilitates the conduct and utilization of research and other scholarly activities. **Evidence 13.3** Provide evidence that nurse researchers are encouraged and enabled to conduct studies; evidence that committees that develop policies and procedures for clinical care base their work on current literature; and evidence that practitioners have easy access to recent literature both within the patient care area and through library and/or online opportunities.	**Force 6.24** Provide evidence that research consultants are actively involved in shaping nursing research infrastructure, capacity, and mentorship.	NK3 Describe and demonstrate that direct-care nurses support the human rights of participants in research protocols.

SOURCES OF EVIDENCE: 2002	SOURCES OF EVIDENCE: 2005	SOURCES OF EVIDENCE: 2008
Criterion 13.4 Advocates for resources to support research. **Evidence:** Provide evidence that adequate, appropriate, and current literature is available to practicing nurses; that nurses are actively encouraged to pursue advanced degrees through tuition or scholarship programs; and the research consultation and assistance are available.	**Force 6.25** Provide a copy of the nursing budget or other sources of funding for the past year, the current year-to-date, and the future projection, highlighting the allocation and utilization of resources for nursing research.	**NK 4** The structure(s) and process(es) used by the organization to develop, expand, and/or advance nursing research.
Criterion 13.5 Promotes research based on knowledge-driven nursing practice. **Evidence:** Provide evidence that research studies have been done or are underway based on findings derived from quality assessment and improvement activities or similar findings.	**Force 6.26** Supply documentation of all nursing research activities that are ongoing, including internal validation studies, internal and external research, and participation in survey completed within the past 12-month period.	**NK4EO** Nursing research studies from the past two (2) years, ongoing or completed, generated from the structure(s) and process(es) in NK4.
	Force 6.27 Provide evidence of education and mentoring activities that have effectively engaged staff nurses in research and/or evidence-based practice activities.	**NK 6** The structure(s) and process(s) used to evaluate existing nursing practice, based on evidence.

continues

TABLE 9.1 *continued*

SOURCES OF EVIDENCE: 2002	SOURCES OF EVIDENCE: 2005	SOURCES OF EVIDENCE: 2008
	Force 6.28 Describe resources available to nursing staff to support participation in nursing research and nursing research utilization activities.	**NK 7** The structure(s) and process(es) used to translate new knowledge into nursing practice.
		NK7EO How translation of new knowledge into nursing practice has affected patient outcomes.

Sources: ANCC Magnet Recognition Program® Application Manuals, 2002, 2005, 2008. ©American Nurses Credentialing Center. All rights reserved. Reproduced with permission of the American Nurses Credentialing Center.

Many varying structures, arrangements, and relationships have been developed to meet the standards for nursing research and research-based practice. Some have established consortia across their states that bring together nurse researchers from school of nursing with clinicians in multiple healthcare settings. Monetary resources and positions to direct and support research have been incorporated into the setting (Urden & Monarch, 2002, p.113). Wilson and colleagues (2013) shared other tactics for practice settings to consider such as lunch and learn sessions on how to critically review a research article, coaching and resources to replicate studies, and the provision of in-services on the IRB and the protection of human subjects.

Of note is the factor that all organizations are facing financial challenges. It is imperative that nurse leaders promote creative and cost-effective strategies to engage nurses in research in the practice settings. Drenkard (2013, p. 246) cites the following ideas:

- Are there university faculty researchers who need partners in the clinical setting?

- Is there a way to align a practicum project for doctorate of nursing practice students from local nursing schools with building the capacity of your organization to conduct and disseminate nursing research?

- Can you hire a PhD researcher part-time to education and support nursing research council members?

- Can you work with your foundation to identify donors whose interests match the areas of clinical research and to solicit funding for nursing research projects?

- Can you form a collegial partnership with hospitals or organizations to share research resources?

- Are there grants you might quality for?

MGH's Magnet® Journey

Similar to the evolution of the emphasis on research and evidence-based practice in the Magnet® Sources of Evidence over the years, the infrastructure and initiatives to realize those requirements have evolved in the practice setting at Massachusetts General Hospital (MGH). In 2003, the ANCC designated MGH as the first Magnet-recogized organization in Massachusetts, and redesignated it in 2007 and 2013.

A knowledge-based commitment to nursing research has long been a part of efforts at MGH (Ives Erickson, 2012). As noted in Chapter 1, "Creating a Culture of Inquiry Within a Healthcare Medical Center," it has taken several decades to cultivate our current culture of inquiry, which started with seeding simple initiatives such as journal clubs, a nursing research committee that facilitated the translation of research into practice, and awarding small research grants to staff with mentorship to address their research questions. The organization's investment in nursing research was formalized with a dedicated research center, the Yvonne L. Munn Center for Nursing Research (Munn Center) (Chapter 3, "Promoting Nursing Research Through the Yvonne L. Munn

Center"), which is part of the larger Institute for Patient Care (Chapter 2 "Creating an Infrastructure that Enhances Professional Practice and Patient Care Services"). Strategies to promote the conduct of research, translation of evidence into practice, and the advancement of innovation are presented in Chapter 3, Chapter 4, "Using, Evaluating, and Integrating an Evidence-Based Practice," and Chapter 5, "Supporting Operational Effectiveness and Encouraging Research Through Innovation," respectively.

In the pages that follow, excerpts from MGH's 2012 Magnet Recognition Program® application submission will illustrate knowledge generation and knowledge translation into practice.

Knowledge Generation

You can review two examples of knowledge generation through the coordination of research efforts by the Munn Center in Appendix A, IRB-Approved Nursing Research Study titled "The Evaluation of an Education Intervention to Enhance Nurses' Skills, Confidence, and Attitudes of Evidence-Based Practice (Grant Funded)," and Appendix B, IRB-Approved Nursing Research study titled "The Impact of Death and Dying in the Intensive Care Unit on New Graduate Nurses (Munn Award)."

Knowledge Translation

At MGH, generating, identifying, and translating new and emerging knowledge are at the core of our four-pronged mission as an academic medical center: practice, education, research, and community. The exponential rate of new biomedical knowledge discovery is ever growing worldwide (Hey, Tansley, & Tolle, 2009). Keeping up with new knowledge is an ongoing challenge that requires a higher level of sophistication than ever before. Zimmermann (2013, p. 371) notes that "if nurses are to possess the capabilities to manage in complex systems, they must be educated in systems theory and the frameworks for translation of new knowledge to practice."

Traditional strategies for broad knowledge translation are described throughout this book and include educational activities of the Norman Knight Nursing Center for Clinical & Professional Development (Chapter 2), the translational activities of the Collaborative Governance Quality and Practice Oversight Committee, the translational research activities of Munn Center (Chapter 3), and the evidence-based, patient education activities of the Blum Patient and Family Learning Center (Chapter 2).

In addition, a number of *new* or *expanding* structures and processes to translate knowledge into practice have been implemented and are highlighted in this section. They are knowledge translation through the following:

- Excellence Every Day Portal

- Innovation units

- Collaborative governance champions

- Interdisciplinary teams

Knowledge Translation Through Excellence Every Day Portal

At MGH, *excellence every day* means striving to provide the best possible care to every patient and family in every moment of every day. It is our philosophy and our commitment.

In an effort to synergize communication and resources, the PCS Excellence Every Day Portal was launched on July 20, 2011 to serve as a central clearinghouse for information related to collaborative governance, Magnet® recognition, and regulatory readiness (http://www.mghpcs.org/EED). The Excellence Every Day Portal (see Figure 9.2), or EED Portal, as it is called, is readily accessible from several routes and provides a new evidence-based focus monthly.

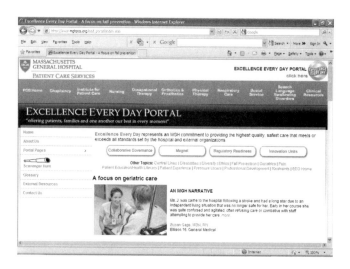

FIGURE 9.2

Excellence Every Day Portal

The EED Portal has become an example of a methodology for successful knowledge translation, an innovation containing just-in-time knowledge with a far reach. Originally marketed as "a link to all things quality and safety," the EED Portal continues to expand with new, updated, easy-to-find content. Consistent with the goal of translating knowledge into practice, the EED Portal has evolved into the destination for information about key topics in clinical practice. It now contains clinical knowledge for practice about central lines, disabilities, diversity, ethics, fall prevention, pain, patient education/health literacy, patient experience, pressure ulcers, and restraints, as well as an expanding "glossary." Each is updated by subject matter experts on an ongoing basis. Key topics (e.g., those related to nursing quality indicators) are annually revisited PCS-wide.

Knowledge Translation Through the Innovation Units

The "innovation units," originally 12 patient care units involved in a pilot project, are serving as the testing ground for innovations in new models and processes of care. The innovation units originated from the need to make care more effective, efficient, and affordable for patients and families.

Over a very short period, the chief nursing officer (CNO) challenged nurses on the inpatient units to embark on this project. Adventurous and inquisitive self-selected nursing leaders jumped on board, despite not fully knowing what was involved.

Interested nursing directors, clinical nurse specialists, and staff nurses wrote one proposal per unit early in the process, identifying at least one innovation that they would implement specific to their units. Over the course of several months, leaders in PCS examined a variety of evidence-based innovations that would assist units in meeting the preselected goals. They selected 15 for implementation on the units (refer to Chapter 5, Figure 5.2 and Table 5.1). The interventions are evidence-based. They were derived from process improvement literature as promising evidence-based interventions specifically designed to improve clinical outcomes, enhance patient- and staff-satisfaction, and reduce costs and lengths of stay. The interventions were vetted with staff during thought-provoking discussions at retreats, breakout sessions, and conversations. Utilizing the EED Portal as the point of knowledge, all the information for and about innovation units can be found there, as well (http://www.mghpcs.org/Innovation_Units/index.asp).

The innovation units are a proving ground for knowledge translation. A comprehensive evaluation is being conducted, specifically examining fidelity and barriers to adoption of the various components. External consultant Marita Titler, PhD, RN, FAAN, a specialist in implementation science and author of the *Translational Research Model*, advocates for piloting and evaluating new EBPs to know whether the intervention will be successful in a particular environment. In essence, the innovation units are implementing "bundles" of evidence-based interventions by using rapid-cycle change. The innovation units are a novel way to translate evidence into practice. Interventions "that work" are disseminated to the other units in the hospital.

Knowledge Translation Through Collaborative Governance Champions

Collaborative governance (CG), our communication and decision-making model, aligns its work to meet the evolving needs of patients and families and the changing healthcare environment. CG plays a pivotal role in the translation of new knowledge into practice.

An often quoted statement about knowledge translation is that it takes, on average, 17 years for new knowledge to go from bench to bedside (Balas & Boren, 2000, p. 65–70). The goal, however, is to quickly put evidence into practice, where it can help patients and families. As new knowledge is translated into practice guidelines, policies, and procedures, the challenge is to make frontline nurses aware of new knowledge as quickly and effectively as possible.

The Champion Model has accelerated the pace of translation. Previously associated with the MGH's Magnet Recognition Program® and Excellence Every Day initiatives, the Champion Model became an integral part of the CG redesign. The Champion Model provides frontline staff with the authority and accountability for conveying key information to their colleagues. The CNO states, "The word champion, versus member, better reflects the evolution of committee members into the empowered communicators, content experts, and leaders they have become" (Ives Erickson, 2011). In fact, those who participate in CG derive a higher level of meaning and competence from their experiences.

According to the Translational Research Model (Titler, 2008), the adoption of new knowledge into practice depends on the characteristics of the innovation and how the innovation is communicated to end users within an organization champions on the Staff Nurse Advisory Committee value their monthly meetings with the CNO. Evaluation reveals that they feel privileged to have early access to information and take their roles as communicators seriously. One Champion shared, "It feels very empowering to explain to staff the innovations being trialed and the reasoning behind them."

Along the same topic, CG Champions accelerate adoption of new knowledge because they are the ones communicating the knowledge to their peers. Similarly, through two-way communication, other members of the organization are educated by the experiences of frontline staff.

One example in 2012 relates to clinical nurses and other clinicians questioning the accuracy of the temporal artery thermometers. Two internal content experts visited the Policies, Procedures, and Products Subcommittee and the Staff Nurse Advisory Committee meetings to clarify some misunderstandings around the programmed settings and use of the temporal artery thermometers. Based on a thorough review of the literature that was conducted by EBP mentors, the experts confirmed the reliability of the thermometers in normothermic and hypothermic patients. The experts then informed the Champions that a research study was planned to evaluate the thermometer's accuracy in hyperthermic patients. Thus, the champions were able to report to their colleagues with new and accurate information about the issues relating to the thermometers and what was being done.

CG committee meetings are a testing ground for new ideas, often raised by frontline clinical nurses, who seek the latest evidence to guide decision-making. The Champions have an increasing responsibility to be evidence communicators to their colleagues on their units. To increase their knowledge of evidence-based decision-making, ongoing educational sessions about EBP are held to introduce the Champions to the concepts of EBP as they relate to their work in CG.

The members of the Research and Evidence-Based Practice Committee utilize several strategies to share research findings to promote their integration into practice. One example is the "Did You Know?" poster series. Figure 9.3 and Figure 9.4 show examples of posters that inform this series.

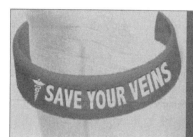

"Save the Veins"
Vein Sparing for patients with renal dysfunction

A Did You Know? poster by
Mary Sylvia-Reardon, RN, DNP Nursing Director of Hemodialysis Unit

TOPIC OF INTEREST

- The use of venous access devices requiring placement in both central and peripheral veins has become prevalent in modern medicine.

- Peripherally inserted central catheters (PICCs) are vascular access devices that can be inserted through a peripheral vein with the tip terminating in the central vascular system.

- Such catheters are inserted through an antecubital vein by needle puncture (Hertzog & Waybill, 2008).

INTRODUCTION

In many institutions, PICCs replace neck or chest wall central venous catheters as the access of choice for intermediate and long term intravenous therapy (Gonsalves et al., 2003). Larger populations of patients receive these lines, not only for in-hospital use, but home therapy as well (Allen et al., 2000).

A survey tool was developed to identify the nursing knowledge and current clinical practice of the PICC-certified members of the MGH IV Therapy Team related to the patient with renal insufficiency. The information gained from the responses identified a need for education. This is a beginning step in the reduction of the number of PICCs placed in this patient population. IRB Protocol #:2009P000865; SRH

In discussions with the Nephrologists at MGH, there was evidence of hemodialysis patients having PICC placement that oftentimes could have been avoided.

REVIEW OF LITERATURE

The literature revealed factors that contribute significantly to damage of upper extremity vessels:

- diameter, location and composition of the catheters
- presence of disease processes
- infusion solutions
- vein choice
- greater incidence of thrombosis in the presence of chemotherapeutic agents
- Lack of radiological visualization

IMPORTANCE OF AVOIDING PICC LINES IN PATIENTS WITH RENAL FAILURE

- Peripherally inserted central catheters (PICC) have become an essential component in the management of increasing numbers of patients, including patients who require hemodialysis or may, in the future require hemodialysis as a result of renal insufficiency (Allen, 2000).

- Complications from central venous catheters (i.e.septicemia, stenosis, thrombosis) often prevent an optimal vascular access that is critical in this population.

GUIDELINES FOR UPPER EXTREMITY VEIN SPARING

- According to the National Kidney Foundation, veins in both arms could potentially be needed for creation of vascular access at some point in time and must be preserved (National Kidney Foundation [NKF], 2006).

- Due to the large number of End Stage Renal Disease patients receiving hemodialysis, as well as peritoneal dialysis and transplant patients who may require hemodialysis at some point, the need for preservation of upper limb vessels is imperative.

- Arm veins suitable for vascular access placement should be preserved regardless of arm dominance. The cephalic veins of the dominant arm should not be used for either venipuncture or intravenous catheters (NKF, 2006).

The MGH Hemodialysis unit adheres to the NKF-Kidney Disease Outcome Quality Initiative (KDOQI) Clinical Practice Guidelines.

GUIDELINES FOR VENOUS ACCESS IN PATIENTS WITH CHRONIC KIDNEY DISEASE OR RENAL INSUFFICIENCY

Identify –
HD patients, present or future
- CKD stages 3,4 or 5, including current stage 5 patients receiving hemodialysis, peritoneal dialysis or transplant patients

Plan –
venous access for stages 3-5

Choose –
- dorsal hand veins for phlebotomy
- proximal peripheral venous access if necessary
- internal jugular veins are preferred for central venous access
- external jugular veins are acceptable alternative

Avoid –
- the subclavian veins

National Kidney Foundation, 2006

FIGURE 9.3

"Did You Know?" poster: Save the Veins

Upper Extremity Veins are the "Lifeline" for patients with End Stage Renal Disease.

As clinicians, we have been charged with the care and preservation of these vessels

OUR PATIENTS' LIVES DEPEND ON IT!!

WHY IS VEIN SPARING IMPORTANT IN PATIENTS WITH RENAL FAILURE?

- Every patient starts with only four superficial upper extremity veins and two subclavian veins

- Avoiding unnecessary iatrogenic trauma to the upper extremity veins is critical for arterio-venous fistula (AVF) creation.

- Not only are the upper extremity veins critical for the creation of the vascular access, but a healthy venous circuit back to the heart is of equal importance.

THROMBOSIS FOLLOWING PICC PLACEMENT

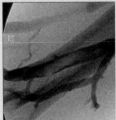

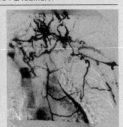

Figure 1

A 38-year-old asymptomatic woman 1 day after PICC placement with inadvertent removal. Venography demonstrates non-occlusive thrombus in a brachial vein.

Printed with author's permission.

Allen et. al., JIVR, 2000

Figure 2

A 9-year-old girl with acute lymphocytic leukemia. Initial left upper extremity venography 1 year ago was normal. Follow-up venography after basic and cephalic PICC placements demonstrated occulsuion of these veins, with occlusion of the central venous system and multiple collaterals. No other form of central venous access had been performed.

A "SAVE THE VEINS" INITIATIVE IS BEING INSTITUTED BY THE HEMODIALYSIS UNIT AND RENAL DIVISION AT THE MGH.

If you are caring for a patient who is wearing a "Save Your Veins" band or you know your patient has renal dysfunction.

Please:

- Contact the patient's Nephrologist or the Access Coordinator prior to PICC placement

- Avoid antecubital punctures whenever possible

- Perform venipuncture below the wrist for blood draws.

- Contact the MGH Hemodialysis Unit 617-726-3700 if you have any questions

REFERENCES

Allen A.W., et.al (2000). Venous thrombosis associated with the placement of peripherally inserted central catheters. Journal of Vascular & Interventional Radiology, 11(10), 1309-14.

Hertzog, D.R. & Waybill, P.N. (2008). Complications and controversies associated with peripherally inserted central catheters. Journal of Infusion Nursing, 31(3), 159-63.

Gonsalves C.F., et al (2003). Incidence of central vein stenosis and occlusion following upper extremity PICC and port placement. Cardiovascular & Interventional Radiology, 26(2), 123-127.

National Kidney Foundation (NKF), (2006).Clinical practice guidelines and clinical practice recommendations. Retrieved August 25, 2008 from http://www.kidney.org/PROFESSIONALS/kdoqi/guideline.

www.mghpcs.org/IPC/Programs/Committees/Research.asp • March 2011

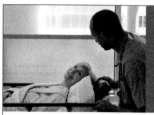

Transporting Patients on Isolation Precautions

What do you mean I shouldn't wear gloves around the hospital?

A Did You Know? poster by Heidi Schleicher, RN, BSN, CIC

WHAT ARE ISOLATION PRECAUTIONS AND WHY DO WE USE THEM?

ISOLATION OF PATIENTS in U.S. hospitals goes back as far as 1877 when patients with infectious diseases were placed in separate facilities known as infectious disease hospitals. In the century to follow many different practices were used to prevent transmission of infection from person to person. In 1985 "Universal Precautions" were introduced in response to the HIV virus with the focus to protect healthcare workers (HCW). Gowns and gloves or "personal protective equipment" (PPE) to prevent exposure to blood-borne pathogens became the norm.

As a result, many began to routinely wear PPE. However, hand hygiene practice suffered as HCWs mistakenly thought gloves were a substitute for hand hygiene. In response, in 1996 the Centers for Disease Control (CDC) dropped "Universal Precautions" and published new guidelines for all patient care known as Standard Precautions. Transmission-based Precautions were added to provide disease or organism-specific isolation guidance.

Standard Precautions protect HCWs from blood-borne pathogens and prevent transmission of infection between patients. They require HCWs to use PPE when contact with blood, body fluids, secretions, excretions, broken skin or mucous membranes is anticipated. PPE is removed when the task is complete. Standard Precautions requires hand hygiene before and after every patient contact or contact with contaminated or potentially contaminated surfaces, regardless of glove use. Disinfection of equipment between patient uses is required. Standard Precautions are required for all patients regardless of whether they have been identified as having an infection. It is the primary strategy today to prevent healthcare-associated infections.

Transmission-based Precautions prevent the transmission of highly transmissible or epidemiologically important pathogens. They are based on the way the organism is spread or the "mode of transmission."[2] The process by which a pathogen "infects" a patient is shown in this "Chain of Infection" diagram.[4]

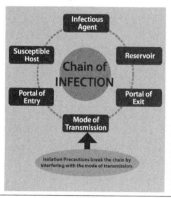

"Transmission-based" Precaution practices interrupt this chain. For example, the flu virus is spread via *droplets* from a cough or sneeze of an infected person. HCWs wear a mask on entry to the room of a patient on Droplet Precautions and the patient *wears a surgical mask during transport.*

Airborne pathogens are very small and may remain suspended in air for long periods. Tuberculosis (TB) is an example of this where TB microorganisms spread from the infected person during talking, sneezing, or coughing. HCWs wear an N-95 respirator in the patient room and the patient on Airborne Precautions *wears a surgical mask for transport.*

Pathogens that are spread by *direct or indirect contact* can be carried from patient to patient via HCWs hands or clothing, or by contaminated equipment (e.g. stethoscopes). Enhanced cleaning of the hospital environment, meticulous hand hygiene, and consistent, correct use of PPE are critical to prevent the spread of these pathogens. Examples are: Methicillin-resistant *Staphylococcus aureus* (MRSA), Vancomycin-resistant *enterococcus* (VRE), and *Clostridium difficile (C. difficile)*. Studies found that MRSA, VRE, and *C. difficile* can survive days to weeks on surfaces. A study from Brigham and Women's Hospital found a 40 percent increased odds of transmission of MRSA or VRE when the prior room occupants were infected with these pathogens despite room cleaning methods that exceeded national standards[5]. Contaminated surfaces can contribute to the spread of these pathogens from HCW hands and/or gloves to patients[3].

Following Contact Precautions correctly while caring for and transporting these patients is critical to limiting contamination. Gowns and gloves are worn while providing care to prevent contamination of hands and clothing, so it is important not to wear PPE in public hallways or spaces during transport. Instead, pushing surfaces should be disinfected, PPE should be removed and hand hygiene should be used to allow for safe transport with clean hands.

FIGURE 9.4

"Did You Know?" poster: Transporting Patients on Isolation Precautions

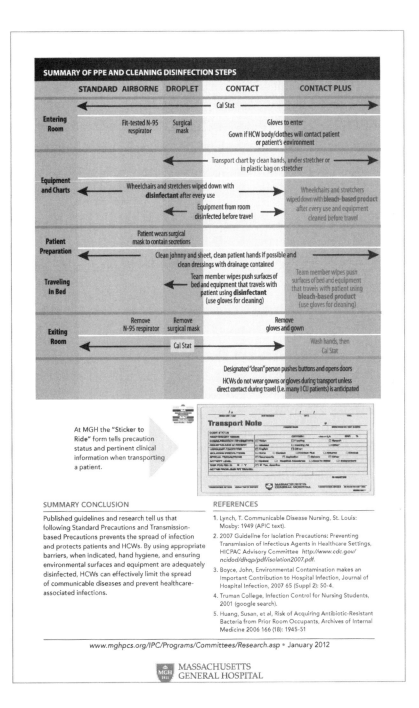

SUMMARY OF PPE AND CLEANING DISINFECTION STEPS

	STANDARD	AIRBORNE	DROPLET	CONTACT	CONTACT PLUS
	← Cal Stat →				
Entering Room		Fit-tested N-95 respirator	Surgical mask	Gloves to enter Gown if HCW body/clothes will contact patient or patient's environment	
		← Transport chart by clean hands, under stretcher or in plastic bag on stretcher →			
Equipment and Charts	← Wheelchairs and stretchers wiped down with **disinfectant** after every use →				Wheelchairs and stretchers wiped down with bleach-based product after every use and equipment cleaned before travel
				← Equipment from room disinfected before travel →	
Patient Preparation		Patient wears surgical mask to contain secretions			
	← Clean johnny and sheet, clean patient hands if possible and clean dressings with drainage contained →				
Traveling in Bed			← Team member wipes push surfaces of bed and equipment that travels with patient using **disinfectant** (use gloves for cleaning)		Team member wipes push surfaces of bed and equipment that travels with patient using bleach-based product (use gloves for cleaning)
Exiting Room		Remove N-95 respirator	Remove surgical mask	Remove gloves and gown	
	← Cal Stat →				Wash hands, then Cal Stat
			Designated "clean" person pushes buttons and opens doors HCWs do not wear gowns or gloves during transport unless direct contact during travel (i.e. many ICU patients) is anticipated		

At MGH the "Sticker to Ride" form tells precaution status and pertinent clinical information when transporting a patient.

Transport Note

SUMMARY CONCLUSION

Published guidelines and research tell us that following Standard Precautions and Transmission-based Precautions prevents the spread of infection and protects patients and HCWs. By using appropriate barriers, when indicated, hand hygiene, and ensuring environmental surfaces and equipment are adequately disinfected, HCWs can effectively limit the spread of communicable diseases and prevent healthcare-associated infections.

REFERENCES

1. Lynch, T. Communicable Disease Nursing, St. Louis: Mosby: 1949 (APIC text).

2. 2007 Guideline for Isolation Precautions: Preventing Transmission of Infectious Agents in Healthcare Settings, HICPAC Advisory Committee http://www.cdc.gov/ncidod/dhqp/pdf/isolation2007.pdf.

3. Boyce, John, Environmental Contamination makes an Important Contribution to Hospital Infection, Journal of Hospital Infection, 2007 65 (Suppl 2): 50-4.

4. Truman College, Infection Control for Nursing Students, 2001 (google search).

5. Huang, Susan, et al, Risk of Acquiring Antibiotic-Resistant Bacteria from Prior Room Occupants, Archives of Internal Medicine 2006 166 (18): 1945-51

www.mghpcs.org/IPC/Programs/Committees/Research.asp • January 2012

MASSACHUSETTS GENERAL HOSPITAL

Knowledge Translation Through Interdisciplinary Teams

At MGH, nurses are encouraged to take leading roles in the translation of new knowledge into practice to improve patient outcomes, not only by their nursing colleagues but also with the interdisciplinary team. Appendix C, "Example of Translation of Evidence into Practice Through Interdisciplinary Teams," describes an example led by Janet Madden, RN, MS, CCNS, clinical nurse specialist in the Newborn Intensive Care Unit at Massachusetts General Hospital *for* Children (MGHfC). The team reduced the prevalence of retinopathy of prematurity (ROP) from 43.2% in 2006 to less than 10% in 2012 through a series of interprofessional interventions. And, in an important final step, Janet disseminated this knowledge to colleagues in an additional translational activity by publishing a manuscript in *Advances in Neonatal Care* (Madden & Bobola, 2010).

Summary

One of the key themes that arose during The Magnet® Listening Tour that newly appointed Magnet Recognition Program® Director Linda Lewis conducted in 2013 was the continued need for Magnet to set the standard for nursing and patient care (Lewis, 2014, p. 496). This is hardwired into the Magnet vision that was defined by the Commission on Magnet® Recognition in 2008:

> *"Magnet® organizations will serve as the fount of knowledge and expertise for the delivery of nursing care globally. They will be solidly grounded in core Magnet principles, flexible and constantly striving for discovery and innovation. They will lead the reformation of health care; the discipline of nursing; and care of the patient, family, and community."*

References

Aiken, L. H. (1981). Nursing priorities for the 1980s: Hospital and nursing homes. *American Journal of Nursing, 81*(2), 324-330.

American Nurses Credentialing Center (ANCC). (2002). *Magnet Recognition Program™: Recognizing Excellence in Nursing Service Health Care Organization Instructions and Application Process Manual.* Washington DC, American Nurses Credentialing Center.

American Nurses Credentialing Center (ANCC). (2004). *Magnet Recognition Program®: Recognizing Excellence in Nursing Services Application Manual 2005.* Washington DC, American Nurses Credentialing Center.

American Nurses Credentialing Center (ANCC). (2008). *Recognizing Nursing Excellence: Magnet Recognition Program® Application Manual.* Washington, DC, American Nurses Credentialing Center.

American Nurses Credentialing Center (ANCC). (2014). *2014 Magnet® Application Manual.* Washington DC, American Nurses Credentialing Center.

American Nurses Credentialing Center Magnet® Model. Retrieved from www.nursecredentialing.org/magnet/programoverview/new-magnet-model.

American Nurses Association (ANA). (1995). *Scope and Standards for Nurse Administrators.* Washington DC, American Nurses Publishing.

American Nurses Association (ANA). (2001b). *Code of Ethics for Nurses with Interpretive Statements.* Washington DC, American Nurses Publishing.

American Nurses Association (ANA). (2003). *Nursing's Social Policy Statement, Second edition.* Washington DC, nursebooks.org.

American Nurses Association (ANA). (2004b). *Scope and Standards for Nurse Administrators, Second Edition,* Washington DC, nursebooks.org.

Balas, E. A., & Boran, S. A. (2000). Managing clinical knowledge for healthcare improvements. In J. Bemmel & A. T. McCray (Eds.), *Yearbook of Medical Informatics* (pp. 65-70). Stuttgart, Germany: Schaltauer.

Drenkard, K. (2013). Creating a culture for advancing nursing research. *Journal of Nursing Administration, 43*(5), 245-246.

Hey, T., Tansley, S., & Tolle, K. (Eds). (2009). *The fourth paradigm: Data-intensive scientific discovery,* Microsoft Research.

Ives Erickson, J. (2011). Collaborative governance re-design. *Caring Headlines,* April 22.

Ives Erickson, J. (2012). 200 years of nursing: A chief nurse's reflections on practice, theory, policy, education, and research. *Journal of Nursing Administration, 42*(1), 9-11.

Lewis, L. (2014). Magnet® Listening Tour 2013-2014. *Journal of Nursing Administration, 44*(10), 495-496.

Luzinski, C. (2012). Advancing the science of nursing, improving the quality of care. *Journal of Nursing Administration, 42*(3), 123-124.

Madden, J. E., & Bobola, D. L. (2010). A data-driven approach to retinopathy of prematurity prevention leads to dramatic change. *Advances in Neonatal Care, 10*(4), 182-187.

McClure, M. L., & Hinshaw, A. S. (2002). *Magnet® hospitals revisited: Attraction and retention of professional nurses.* American Academy of Nursing. Washington, DC: American Nurses Publishing.

McClure, M. L., Poulin, M. A., Sovie, M. D., & Wandelt, M. A. (1983). *Magnet® hospitals: Attraction and retention of professional nurses.* Kansas City, MO: American Nurses Association.

Titler, M. (2008). *The evidence for evidence-based practice implementation. In R. Hughes (Ed.), Patient safety and quality: An evidence-based handbook for nurses.* (AHRQ Publication No. 08 0043). Rockville, MD. Agency for Healthcare Research and Quality. Retrieved from http://www.ncbi.nlm.nih.gov/books/NBK2659/.

Urden, L. D., & Monarch, K. (2002). *The ANCC Magnet Recognition Program: Converting research findings into action* (pp. 103–116). In M. K. McClure & A. S. Hinshaw (Eds.), *Magnet® hospitals revisited: Attraction and retention of professional nurses.* Washington, DC: American Nurses Publishing.

Wilson, B., Kelly, L., Reifsnider, E., Pipe, T., & Brumfield, B. (2013). *Journal of Nursing Administration, 43*(2).

Zimmermann, D. (2013). An essential next step for nursing. *Journal of Nursing Administration, 43*(7/8).

Chapter 10
Concluding Thoughts

–Jeanette Ives Erickson, DNP, RN, NEA-BC, FAAN
–Dorothy A. Jones, EdD, RN, FAAN, FNI
–Marianne Ditomassi, DNP, MBA, RN

"Guided by the needs of our patients and their families, we aim to deliver the very best health care in a safe, compassionate environment; to advance that care through innovative research and education; and to improve the health and well-being of the diverse communities we serve."

–Mission Statement, Massachusetts General Hospital

"Nursing research provides the scientific basis for the practice of the profession" (AACN, 2012, p. 1). It is often grounded in a variety of theoretical frameworks and methodological approaches, and its focus centers on the health and well-being of society. Core to the development and sustainability of a nursing research program within a clinical practice environment is the alignment of a research agenda with the mission and values of the organization and the organizational and nursing service strategic plan. The vision and strategy of nursing research within this framework is linked to the belief that knowledge is constantly being built and expanded through research.

"It is the general conception that any field of inquiry determines the kind of knowledge that field aims to develop as well as the manner in which that knowledge is to be organized, tested, applied" (Carper, 1978, p. 13). Within the practice environment, the development of a nursing research agenda is a cooperative journey involving nurse scientists, administrators, clinical nurses, patients, and families. This coalition, along with the support and resources needed to fund research and inquiry, help create the culture that can build, test, and translate nursing knowledge to inform practice and guide inquiry for the advancement of the discipline and the betterment of society.

Knowledge Development: An Iterative Process

The journey of nursing research is about knowledge development, its use, and its translation into care redesign. Knowledge development is an iterative process (see Figure 10.1). The process can begin by identifying gaps in knowledge, raising new questions in practice, challenging existing evidence, or using new methodological approaches to answer new challenges in care delivery.

For example, when questions are raised within practice, the process looks like this:

1. Nurses look to available resources for evidence.

2. When this information is not available, a gap in knowledge is identified and research inquiry begins.

3. To answer these new questions or hypotheses, the literature is reviewed, a methodology is developed, and the investigation is launched by an individual researcher or team.

4. The resulting knowledge (evidence) is then evaluated, validated, and/or refined and used (translated) to enhance cost-effective, safe, high-quality, efficient patient/family/community-centric care (IOM, 2010).

Over time, new questions arise, and nursing science evolves and expands.

Research is part of an iterative process.
We cannot have one without the other.

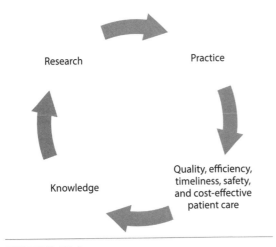

FIGURE 10.1

Knowledge development: An iterative process

What it means is that knowledge development can begin in practice, with a practice issue, or be generated and tested as a theoretical worldview or emerge as a research question. The ultimate result is new information is added to our knowledge and can guide practice, improve quality and safety, foster cost effectiveness, and enhance patient/family centric care. The generation of a new hypothesis will promote inquiry, new investigation, and translation of new knowledge to improve patient/family centric care. Whenever we engage in discovery, we are impacting knowledge development, patient care, and uncovering science.

The Yvonne L. Munn Center for Nursing: Central to Facilitating the Process of Discovery

At the Massachusetts General Hospital (MGH), The Yvonne L Munn Center for Nursing Research (Munn Center) is a thriving and vital part of the Department of Nursing, Patient Care Services (PCS), and the entire organization. During its tenure, the center's leadership, as well as nurse scientists, have guided clinical nurses as they solved dilemmas in practice, redesigned care delivery, measured the impact of creative interventions, fostered innovations, and promoted a practice environment that values inquiry and discovery. Within the Munn Center at MGH, all nurses, especially nurse researchers/scientists, are positioned to address the concerns of providers and patients to generate, test, and refine knowledge that will lead to care redesign and impact care at the bedside, in community health centers, in global health programs, in industry, and in patients' homes.

Munn Center: Leveraging the Potential of Nursing Knowledge

As changes in healthcare evolve, nursing research is the important lynchpin between current practice and the discovery of new ways to improve the health of individuals, families, and populations within communities served. The development of a research center that advances a nursing research agenda within a multidisciplinary practice environment is an ambitious commitment. It is predicated on the valuing of nursing knowledge and its potential to promote excellence in patient care and advancing cross-discipline collaboration.

Fostering an environment of discovery that accelerates patient care must be the driving force that guides the work. The focus needs to be on creating improvements in the promotion of health for all and the management of patients' response to illness. Nurse researchers within the practice setting have a unique opportunity to develop a research agenda that complements the strategic goals of the organization; improves care at the bedside; enhances the use of technology; introduces new patient/family-centric, nurse-designed care delivery models; and creates a practice environment that uncovers new knowledge embedded in the patient/family healthcare experience.

Munn Center: Impact So Far

The impact of the Munn Center has been realized in many ways, including:

- The development of an infrastructure to advance nursing research and collaborate with other scientists

- Integration of nursing research, inquiry, evidence, and discovery into the culture of care at MGH

- Advancement of a nursing research agenda that focuses on the following:

  - The care of the older adult

  - Palliative and end-of-life care

  - Women's health (especially in vulnerable populations)

  - Interventions that foster growth and development in children (especially premature infants and nutritional innovation)

  - Reducing instances of hospital-acquired infections, pressure ulcers, and falls

  - Using new technology to enhance patient monitoring

  - Promoting patient comfort through complementary healing interventions

  - Enhancing nurses' knowledge regarding patient decision-making and resolving ethical conflict

  - Evaluating innovation effectiveness and implementation and evaluation of a professional practice model

- Expansion of opportunities for all nurses to engage in research

- Establishment of new partnerships, multidisciplinary collaborations, and clinical investigation with researchers at MGH and around the globe

- Obtainment of national research funding

- Recognition of nursing research as a contributor to the overall MGH research enterprise

- Dissemination of nursing research findings through global presentations and in the international literature

These outcomes, along with initiating interest in professional advancement and generating the largest cohort of doctorally prepared nurse researchers engaged in clinical practice, are a testimony to the accomplishments of the past. As we face our future, new research opportunities and discoveries through team and collaborative investigations are integral to the continued advancement of nursing research and promotion of a scientific agenda of discovery. These efforts will impact professional practice and contribute to the integration of nursing knowledge to guide the development of healthcare delivery systems on a global level.

Moving Nursing Research Forward

Strategically designed structures and settings like the Munn Center have proven to be an innovation to help nurses overcome the barriers linked to advancing an agenda in clinical practice. The environment provides both the infrastructure and support needed to integrate nursing research into the fabric of patient care delivery (Jones, 2012, p. 315).

The development and advancements of the Munn Center are within the context of a large and successful research agenda throughout the organization. "With an annual research budget of more than $786 million, MGH conducts the largest hospital-based research program in the United States—a program that spans more than 20 clinical departments and centers across the hospital. This funding drives discoveries and breakthroughs in basic and clinical research, which translate into new and better treatments that transform medical practice and patient care (MGH, n.d.).

The research strategic plan creates the structure to advance knowledge generation and opportunities for discovery.

"To sustain the professional practice environment requires knowledge and a culture of inquiry. The development, use, and continued refinement of knowledge enable the clinician to bring the best of the discipline forward to advance care" (Ives Erickson, Jones, & Ditomassi, 2013, p. 352).

Awareness of practice or limitations in practice is explicit or implicit. Patricia Benner who taught us that our capacity to know develops by being with our patients best describes knowledge acquisition involving cognitive processes and reasoning. Benner's groundbreaking work *From Novice to Expert* (1984) describes that skill acquisition and knowledge are integral to understanding how one makes advances in clinical practice. Without new knowledge caregivers cannot be responsive to the increasing level of complexity of our patients and care environments. Knowledge informs the plan of care for each patient as individuals, practice standards, and standards of care.

The development of the Munn Center holds a disciplinary responsibility to the Patient Care Services (PCS) division and MGH. Through the vision of nurse leaders, the voice of nursing science has grown outside of an academic setting and within the space of practice. The growth of nursing research can be realized to its fullest only with sustained development and advancement of its scholars. At MGH, the collaborative support of many fosters an environment that can result in new research that will used to improve the health of all people.

Advancing the research agenda initiated at MGH requires the continued advancement of our nurse scientists, funding and resources to support the work, and multidisciplinary collaborations to link nursing knowledge to a broader research agenda. The development of multisite and international studies needs to continue, as we expand our understanding of the impact of illness on recovery or address care transitions including palliative care. The growth of innovative funding opportunities, such as the National Institutes of Health (NIH) Patient-Centered Outcomes Research Institute (PCORI) mechanism, and internal opportunities to consult and collaborate around new funding options will increase the visibility of nursing research and help advance inquiry and make visible the focus of the discipline. "No discipline is more integral and essential within every level of the healthcare delivery system than nursing...it touches the lives of every person at some point in their lives" (Grady, 2011, p. 6).

Summary

As reiterated throughout this book and especially within this chapter, nursing research and the exploitation of the potential for nurses to actively engage in the pursuit of knowledge through inquiry is a reality. Whether in teams or in collaboration with other disciplines, nurse scholars are an integral component for positive advancements made in patient care. Nursing research is a journey, not a destination. Collaborative stakeholders both drive those efforts and derive applicable benefits as nursing research is leveraged for clinical practice/process gains. Continued development of all nurses in the pursuit of discovery enhances the practice environment and the culture of care. Knowledge developed in the process fosters professional development, promotes knowledge-based care and helps achieve cost-effective, safe, high quality patient care outcomes that enrich the human potential and that of our global society.

References

American Association of Colleges of Nursing (AACN). (2012). Position statement on nursing research. Washington, DC: American Association of Colleges of Nursing.

Benner, P. (1984). *From novice to expert: Excellence and power in clinical nursing practice.* Menlo Park, CA: Addison-Wesley.

Carper, B. (1978). Fundamental patterns of knowing in nursing. *Annals of Nursing Science, 1*(1), 13-24.

Grady, P. (2011). Bringing science to life. Bethesda, MD: NIH NINR strategic plan.

Institute of Medicine (IOM). (2010). *The future of nursing: Leading change, advancing health.* Washington, DC: Institute of Medicine.

Ives Erickson, J., Jones, D. A., & Ditomassi, M. (2012). *Fostering nurse-led care: Professional practice for the bedside leader from MGH.* Indianapolis, IN: Sigma Theta Tau.

Jones, D.A. (2012). Realizing the IOM future of nursing research within clinical practice. *Nursing Research, 61*(5), 315.

Massachusetts General Hospital (MGH). (n.d.). Hospital overview. Retrieved from www.massgeneral.org/about/overview.aspx

Appendix A

The Evaluation of an Educational Intervention to Enhance Nurses' Skills, Confidence, and Attitudes of Evidence-Based Practice

(Retooling for Evidence-Based Nursing Practice Grant)

–Diane L. Carroll, PhD, RN, FAAN
–Linda Brandt, RN, MS
–Susan Lee, PhD, RN

(Excerpt from 2012 MGH Magnet Recognition Program® evidence)

1. Purpose and Background:

The purpose of this study was to determine the extent to which a multi-modal educational intervention impacts beliefs, skills, and confidence related to evidence-based practice among nurses at MGH. This study was part of the Retooling for Evidence-Based Nursing Practice Project (REBNP).

In *Crossing the Quality Chasm* (IOM, 2001, pp. 207, 211), the Committee on Quality of Health Care in America stated that, "Americans should be able to count on receiving care that meets their needs and is based on the best scientific knowledge. Yet there is strong evidence that this frequently is not the case." The Committee identified six aims to improve the quality of health care; health care should be safe, effective, patient-centered, timely, efficient, and equitable. Furthermore, the Committee advocated fundamental changes in the preparation of the workforce in order to achieve these aims. Evidence-based practice (EBP) is a critical skill needed by registered nurses to practice in existing and emerging organized health care systems.

Evidence-based practice is defined as the conscientious and judicious use of current best evidence in conjunction with clinical expertise and patient values to guide health care decisions (IOM, 2001; Titler, n.d.). Evidence-based practice has been identified as a national priority for creating a quality health care system and as a core competency required for all health care professionals in the 21st century (Institute of Medicine, 2003). In order for nursing to meet this professional competency, there is a need for continuing education programs that train nurses in effectively finding, critically appraising, and synthesizing evidence in order to identify and apply the best available scientific knowledge for clinical decision-making which will ensure high quality care and decrease healthcare disparities. However, little is known about how to effectively educate nurses in this area, and how to sustain the impact of education after its completion.

The goal of the educational component of the REBNP Project was to develop, implement, and evaluate a sequential, multimodal nursing continuing education program that would teach nurses the core skills of EBP through didactic classes, seminars, workshops, web-based classes, and a practicum for which continuing education credit was provided.

2. Description of Work:

This was a descriptive, repeated measures study. Nurse participants in an educational program, the Clinical Inquiry Institute, were surveyed at Time 1 (baseline), Time 2 (upon completion of program), and Time 3 (4 months after the program), using a confidential, web-based survey. The study was approved by the Partners Human Research Committee; exempt status was granted.

The Clinical Inquiry Institute was a 2-day course offered in May 2010 and May 2011. Marketing materials were emailed to all units and departments in PCS, although clinical nurse specialists were strongly encouraged to attend.

Prior to participating in the Clinical Inquiry Institute, prerequisite self-study materials were distributed. Participants were also required to bring a clinical question, which required additional study on their part. After the Clinical Inquiry Institute, topical seminars were offered biweekly to hone their skills in specific areas. The topical seminars continued for 8 months.

3. Team Membership:

There were 50 participants in the Clinical Inquiry Institute. (Refer to Table A.1 for demographic characteristics of participants.) In the first cohort, 16 nurse leaders including clinical nurse specialists, nursing director, and clinical educators participated. In the second cohort, 34 nurse participants consisting of staff nurses, informatics nurses, nurse practitioners and clinical nurse specialists participated. The majority of the participants were master's-prepared as the time of the institute. Nurses came from a variety of different units in the hospital, including the out-patient areas. Forty-eight completed the surveys.

4. Measurement:

To measure participants' beliefs about EBP, sub-scales from an instrument developed by Nagy, Lumby, McKinley, and Macfarlane and colleagues (Nagy, McKinley, Macfarlane; 2001, pp. 314-321) was used, after receiving permission from the authors. The original instrument was tested in Australia. Nagy and colleagues used qualitative interviews to identify themes from which they developed a set of questions. They distributed the 50-item questionnaire to 1250 nurses with a response of 816 (65%). Each item had a response from 1-strongly disagree to 5-strongly agree. Principal axis factor analysis was used to identify groups of questions to determine underlining factors.

TABLE A.1   Demographic Characteristics of Participants

VARIABLE	(N = 48)	
Age	49.2 ± 10.2 years	
Gender	47 females / 3 males	
Years in Nursing	21 ± 12.9 years	
Years at Academic Medical Center	19.3 ± 12.2 years	
Initial Nursing Education	Diploma	8
	Associate Degree	7
	Bachelor's Degree	17
	Master's Degree	16
Current Position	Clinical Nurse Specialist	20
	Nurse Director	2
	Clinical Educator	4
	Nurse Practitioner	8
	Staff Nurse	6
	Informatics Nurse	7
	Quality Assurance Nurse	1

To measure skills and confidence, the co-investigators used the National Consensus of Essential Competencies for Evidence-Based Practice in Nursing (Stevens, 2005) to identify basic EBP competencies that would be targeted in the educational program. The co-investigators developed the Skills and Confidence Sub-Scale items from these competency statements. Participants were asked to rate their skills and confidence on 10 items using a four-point Likert scale (1 = not at all confident to 4 = extremely confident). The Cronbach's alpha for these scales were 0.83 to 0.87 in this evaluation.

The data were entered into the SPSS statistical package (SPSS v. 15; IBM) for data reduction and scoring to the appropriate sub-scale. The analysis proceeded with descriptive statistics on the demographic data. Cronbach's alpha was computed on all instruments utilized in this study. A repeated measures analysis of variance (ANOVA) was used to compare mean scores between the different measurement Times 1–3. The level of significance was set at $p < 0.05$.

The mean scores on all three Sub-Scales are displayed in Table A.2. Prior to participating in the educational program, participants scored highly on the Beliefs Sub-Scale indicating that they valued the importance of EBP. These scores remained high over time; there was no change in the pre/post scores on this sub-scale. The results of the Skills Sub-Scale at Time 1 indicated that there were opportunities to enhance their skills. The educational intervention significantly enhanced their skills ($p = 0.003$). The mean scores on the Confidence Sub-Scale indicated that, prior to the Clinical Inquiry Institute, 23 (46%) participants had no confidence in being able to perform components of evidence based practice. This significantly changed after the education ($p = 0.000$).

In summary, the Clinical Inquiry Institute did not change participants' beliefs in the value of EBP; this was highly rated both before and after the education. Nurses' skills and confidence practicing from an evidence base significantly increased and remained so, even 4 months later. The findings suggest that the Clinical Inquiry Institute improved nurses' skills and confidence.

The findings also add to what is known about EBP education and will be used to structure future educational programs.

TABLE A.2 Results

SUB-SCALES	TIME 1 PRE-EDUCATION N = 48	TIME 2 POST-EDUCATION N = 44	TIME 3 4 MONTHS POST-EDUCATION N = 37	F	P
Beliefs	4.60 ± 0.33	4.75 ± 0.29	4.66 ± 0.34	0.67	0.43
Skills	3.44 ± 0.33	3.81 ± 0.23	3.74 ± 0.26	11.9	0.003
Confidence*	1.98 ± 0.44	2.64 ± 0.44	2.54 ± 0.46	21.4	0.000

Belief and Skills Sub-Scales were scored from 1-5 (strongly disagree to strongly agree)
*Confidence Sub-Scale scored from 1-4 (not at all confident to totally confident)

References

Institute of Medicine (IOM) (2001). *Crossing the quality chasm: A new health system for the 21st century.* Washington, DC: National Academy Press

Institute of Medicine (IOM) (2003). Committee on the Health Professionals Education Summit. *Health professions education: A bridge to quality.* Washington, DC: National Academies Press.

Nagy, S., Lumby, J., McKinley, S., & Macfarlane, C. (2001). Nurses' beliefs about the conditions that hinder or support evidence-based nursing. *International Journal of Nursing Practice, 7*(5), 314-321.

Stevens, K. R. (2005). *Essential competencies for evidence-based practice in nursing*, (1st ed.). San Antonio, TX: Academic Center for Evidence-Based Practice, UTHSCSA.

Titler, M. (n.d.). Overview of evidence-based practice and research utilization. University of Iowa Hospitals and Clinics. Retrieved from https://icon.uiowa.edu.

Appendix B
Yvonne L. Munn Nursing Research Award Exemplar

The Impact of Death and Dying in the Intensive Care Unit on New Graduate Nurses

–Tara Tehan, MSN, MBA, RN

–Mary Guanci, MSN, RN, CNRN

–Donna Perry, PhD, RN, (mentor)

The annual Yvonne L. Munn Nursing Research Awards (MNRA) provide opportunities for nurses to conduct mentored nursing research projects that will advance nursing knowledge and improve the care of patients and families.

(Excerpt from MGH Magnet Recognition Program® evidence)

1. Purpose and Background

On average, in America's intensive care units (ICU), the mortality rate is between 20–25%, indicating that death is a regular occurrence. As the healthcare providers most present at the bedside, nurses must be comfortable providing care to dying patients and their families. Unfortunately, the new graduate nurse *who begins his/her career in the ICU* may not have prior experience or skills to provide the care needed by patients and grieving families. This study was designed to explore the experiences of new nurses around caring for dying patients and their families. Learning about the experience will help inform leadership practice and guide interventions the nursing leaders can implement around recruitment, education, and support for new nurses.

Literature review

While the experience of new nurses is well described in the literature, there is little research describing the experience of the new graduate nurse in the ICU and his/her experience around death and dying. Therefore, a literature search was conducted on new graduate nurses in non-specialty areas and death and dying related to moral distress, burnout and turnover.

Brisley and Wood (2004) interviewed a group of new graduate nurses and reported the following themes: feelings of fear and anxiety around death, lack of undergraduate preparation, and the need for support. Casey, Fink, Krugman, and Propst found similar results in a study with 270 new graduate nurses, some of which were critical-care nurses. 37% of this sample reported they were uncomfortable caring for dying patients.

Moral distress is defined by Jamestown as a "painful feeling or psychological disequilibrium that occurs in situations in which the ethically right course of action is known but cannot be acted upon." (Jameston, 1984). Moral distress is well described in the literature and the impact on nurses has been documented. In 2004, Mary Corley described a model in which moral distress, moral suffering, and moral residue impacts the patient, nurse and organization (Corley, 2002). The impact on the patient includes increased patient discomfort. Resignation, burnout, and leaving the profession may result when the nurse experiences moral distress. Finally, turnover, decreased quality, and decreased patient satisfaction may be an organizational result. McClendon and Buckner state, "It seemed that nurses experience a high level of moral distress at the beginning of their career, which decreased to a moderate level over time and eventually declined to a low level over a number of years." (McClendon & Buckner, 2007). In this same study involving intensive care and cardiac care nurses, the most frequently encountered situation involved families wishing to continue aggressive treatment when it would not benefit the patient. Meltzer and Huckabay described this same phenomenon and concluded that care perceived as futile or non-beneficial resulted in emotional exhaustion for the nurse (Meltzer & Huckabay, 2004). As technology has advanced, these situations that create moral distress occur more frequently and will be encountered by the new graduate nurse starting his or her career in the ICU. A necessary step in developing interventions to support the nurse is to learn what the experience is like.

Over three decades ago, Benner described the development of the new nurses in *From Novice to Expert* (Benner, 1984). Benner describes the novice nurse as one who "has no experience in the situations in which they are expected to perform." Gradually the nurse moves through five stages: novice, advanced beginner, competent, proficient, and expert. In her 1992 article "From Beginner to Expert: Gaining a Differentiated Clinical World in Critical Care Nurse," Benner states that nurses at different levels of practice differ not only in skill but also in their sense of agency. The advanced beginner questions their own sense of agency and feels an overwhelming sense to perform and responsibility for the patient, "At this point, their responsible action or agency does not often include determining what to do or even how to do it, but rather following what has been designed and structured by others." (Benner, Tanner & Chesla, 1992). Unfortunately the death and dying process cannot be designed or structured, but is determined by each patient and family. Benner's theory will guide the investigators.

This study will add to the knowledge of how graduate nurses who begin their career in the intensive care unit experience care for dying patients. It will also provide information on the gaps that exist in the current orientation and support infrastructure. Developing programs and interventions that assist the nurse in being comfortable and competent in this context will benefit patients and families cared for by new graduate nurses.

2. Description of Work

This study sought to explore the lived experience of the new graduate nurse in the intensive care unit around death and dying through the following research questions:

1. What is the experience of the new graduate nurse as he/she cares for dying patients and their families in the ICU?

2. What impact does the death and dying experience have on the new graduate nurse in the ICU?

3. What education and support structures are needed by new graduate nurses to care for self, the patient, and the family?

This study used Benner's Novice to Expert/Dreyfus Model of Skill Acquisition to frame the research questions. Qualitative methods using a phenomenological approach aimed to explore the lived experience of the nurses.

Participants in the 2010 Critical-Care Program at MGH were recruited to participate in the study. After receiving approval by the Partners Human Subjects Committee, the participants were recruited through email. Eight nurses agreed to participate. Data collection followed.

The investigators conducted a primary interview, during the first 6 months of the critical care nurse residency program, using a flexible interview guide. One follow-up interview, using a similar guide, occurred at 18–27 months into the program. All interviews were audiotaped and transcribed. This was followed by data analysis and synthesis.

3. Team Membership

The study was a nurse-driven investigation and funded by a Munn Nursing Research Award. (MNRA). All participants in the 2010 MGH New Graduate in Critical-Care Program were invited to participate. The study sample comprised eight nurses. This number was deemed sufficient by the mentor for this qualitative study due to its nature as pilot work.

4. Measurement

A nurse scientist who is an expert in qualitative methods mentored the novice co-investigators (PI) in the phenomenological approach. The interview tapes were transcribed by the PIs so that they could become generally familiar with the data. The PIs read the transcripts several times to identify significant statements which illustrated the nurses' experiences. Consistent with common phenomenological data analysis, they developed themes from the statements. The themes that emerged with corresponding supportive data.

The conceptual model (Figure B.1) describes the nurses' pathways in practice related to building confidence in clinical situations involving death and dying. The model was derived from the data, with the assistance of the mentor. The

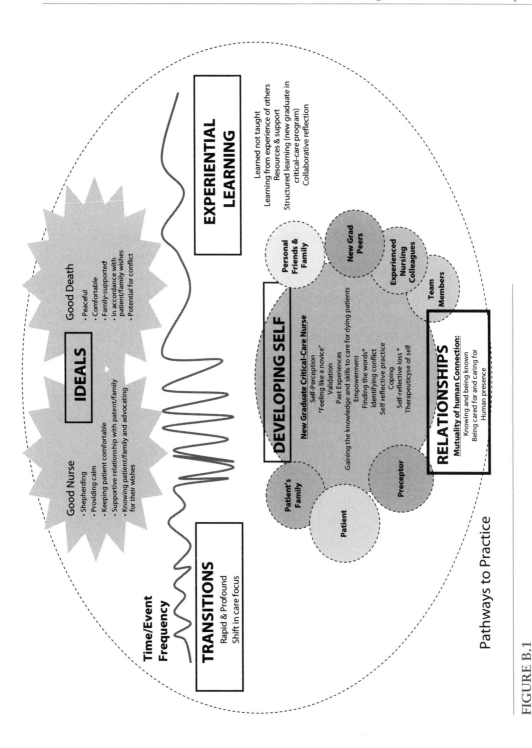

FIGURE B.1

Conceptual Model of Death and Dying as Experiential Learning

nurses reported holding *ideals* about the "good nurse" and his/her role in achieving a "good death" for the patient and family. The nurses report that the rapid and profound *transitions* in patients' conditions are disorienting for them as the focus of care quickly switched to the family who became their new patients. They realized that they were not taught these skills in school but that they were developed *experientially*. Furthermore, clinical experiences with death caused them to reflect on their own beliefs, leading to growth and *development of self*.

The implications for practice focus on better preparation for death and dying for nurses in the New Graduate Critical Care Residency Program. New nurses can be asked in their recruitment interviews about their professional experiences with death and dying in order to assess learning needs. New nurses can be provided with mentored clinical experiences during their orientation so that they care for dying patients while having their preceptors at hand to guide them and to role model. Role-playing conversations with families at end of life and simulating family meetings can develop communication skills and increase nurses' confidence in these areas. Formal supports, such as peer and team de-briefings can be established in the ICUs to provide immediate support. Increasing preceptors' awareness of these findings so that they can be present and attentive to new nurses will enhance the learning. Teaching nurses self-care strategies to improve coping may enhance resilience.

Future research is needed in this area, which could be expanded to new graduates in other critical care residency programs. An instrument designed to assess new graduates' comfort and skill in various domains of practice may be useful in uncovering areas for education. The use of simulation and role play to improve confidence is an area that needs the development of valid and reliable measures. Until that time, nursing leaders can be instrumental on their own units in attending to this very important dimension of human caring.

References

Benner, P. (1984). *From novice to expert: Excellence and power in clinical nursing practice.* Upper Saddle River, NJ: Prentice-Hall.

Benner, P., Tanner, C., & Chesla, C. (1992). From beginner to expert: Gaining a differentiated clinical world in critical care nursing. *Advances in Nursing Science, 14*(3), 13-28.

Brisley, P., & Wood, L. (2004). The impact of education and experience on death anxiety in new graduate nurses. *Contemporary Nurse, 17*(1-2), 102-108.

Casey, K., Fink, R., Krugman, & Propst, J. (2004). The graduate nurse experience. *Journal of Nursing Administration, 34*(6), 303-311.

Corley, M. (2002). Nurse moral distress: A proposed theory and research agenda. *Nursing Ethics, 9*(6), 636-649.

Jameston, A. (1984). *Nursing practice: The ethical issue.* Englewood Cliffs, NJ: Prentice Hall.

McClendon, H. & Buckner, E. (2007). Distressing situations in the intensive care unit: A descriptive study of nurses' responses. *Dimension of Critical Care Nursing, 26*(5), 199-206.

Meltzer, K., & Huckabay, L. (2004). Critical care nurses' perceptions of futile care and its effect on burnout. *American Journal of Critical Care, 13*(3), 202-208.

Appendix C
Example of Translation of Evidence into Practice through Interdisciplinary Teams

Reducing Retinopathy of Prematurity

–*Janet E. Madden, MS, RN, CCNS, Principal Investigator*
–*Deborah L. Bobola, BSN, RN, Clinical Scholar*

(Excerpt from MGH Magnet Recognition Program® evidence)

1. Describe the purpose and background.

The purpose of this performance improvement project was to reduce the prevalence and severity of retinopathy of prematurity (ROP) among a population of infants born at less than or equal to 28 weeks gestation and/or weighing 1,500 grams or less.

Retinopathy of prematurity (ROP) is a common disease of premature infants and the leading cause of childhood blindness in developed countries. In 2006, the MGH for Children (MGHfC) Newborn Intensive Care Unit (NICU) joined the Vermont Oxford Network (VON), a collaboration of health professionals whose work is focused on improving the quality of care for NICU patients and their families. The VON maintains a database that includes information about the care and outcomes of high-risk newborns. Worldwide, more than 800 NICUs are enrolled in the VON. Since 2006, MGH NICU nurses have been able to view their performance against globally benchmarked data.

The data shown in Table C.1, shown as, "MGH 2006," revealed some disappointing information to the NICU Staff. The NICU team learned that in three VON categories, the MGHfC data was higher than average. The categories were "any ROP," "severe ROP," and "ROP requiring surgery," or "Surgical ROP," the latter being twice that of comparable cohorts.

TABLE C.1 Comparison of Prevalence of ROP

	ANY ROP (%)	SEVERE ROP (%)	SURGICAL ROP (%)
MGH 2006	43.2	13.6	9.5
2006 Benchmarks:			
VON	38	8.3	4.4
Massachusetts NICUs	39.9	9.3	5
All US NICUs	40.1	8.8	4.6

Described in this section are the components of the process improvement processes that are ongoing in order to continue to improve metrics as new information becomes available in this area.

2. Describe how the work was done.

The NICU team began by developing a Nursing Practice Guideline which evolved into the ROP Guideline in 2008, and was updated in 2010 and 2011 to ensure continued best evidence. The NICU clinical nurses continue to closely adhere to the ROP Guideline. Over the years, nurses have adjusted practice to embed best practices into the unit's culture. They identify infants meeting criteria and maintain oxygen saturation at desired levels. They continue to create nursing assignments that support clinical nurses at the bedside, providing them with the necessary flexibility to be readily available to intervene and co-manage these patients with the respiratory therapists. The susceptible infants are identified on the whiteboards (location of group report) as well as the cardiac monitor in the infants' rooms. In addition, once an infant matures to 32 weeks gestation, they are examined on a regular schedule by ophthalmologists from the Massachusetts Eye and Ear Infirmary. Each Monday, the resource nurses receive an email identifying which infants will be examined that day. After the exams, the ophthalmologists inform the staff of the exam findings and the exams are discussed at weekly interprofessional rounds. They are aware weekly of each infant's status with respect to his/her eye development. The nurses continue to be vigilant for ways to fine tune these processes.

3. Describe who was involved.

The NICU clinical nurse specialist (CNS) took a lead role in this project. The CNS was joined by a clinical nurse, who is a Clinical Scholar, the highest level a nurse can achieve in the Clinical Recognition Program, our advancement model. The interdisciplinary team, including the nursing director, medical director, and respiratory therapy supervisors, supported adherence to the ROP Guideline to ensure that all members caring for susceptible infants were following the same guideline. The direct care providers involved included all NICU clinical nurses and respiratory therapists.

4. Describe the measurement used to evaluate the outcomes.

The clinical nurses and entire interdisciplinary team monitored the incidence and severity of ROP on a weekly basis after the Ophthalmologists completed their exams. In addition, the data for each infant is submitted to VON and every case of ROP is included in their annual reporting.

Every incidence of ROP was documented by chart abstraction and submitted to the VON network. The earlier reductions in ROP, as described in the article written by the MGH CNS and Clinical Scholar, resulted in the reduction of the incidence of "any ROP" from 43.2% in 2006 to 6% in 2008, a reduction in "severe ROP" from 13.6% in 2006 to 2% in 2008, and a reduction in "surgical ROP" from 9.5% to 2% (Table C.2).

TABLE C.2 Comparison of Prevalence of ROP

	ANY ROP	SEVERE ROP	SURGICAL ROP
MGH 2006	43.2	13.6	9.5
MGH 2008	6	2	2
VON	38	8.3	4.4
2006 Benchmarks:			
Massachusetts NICUs	39.9	9.3	5
All US NICUs	40.1	8.8	4.6

The graph found in Figure C.1 contains the MGHfC NICU and VON ROP rates for the years 2010 through Quarter 2 of 2012. The top graph shows that 100% of newborns at MGHfC are screened for ROP, consistently exceeding the VON benchmark (93.80%) for all eight quarters. The lower graph shows that the prevalence of ROP ranged from 0.00% for four quarters to 8.33%, 11.11%, and 33.33% for one quarter, respectively, while the VON benchmark for 2010 was 43.20%. The rate decreased significantly from Quarter 1 in 2010 from 33.33% to less than 12%. Again, MGHfC consistently exceeded the VON benchmark. Although the intent is to prevent ROP for all infants in the MGHfC NICU, the NICU team believes that the interventions in place supported and sustained the gains in reducing the incidence and severity of ROP in the NICU.

Massachusetts General Hospital
Patient Care Services Office of Quality and Safety
Neonatal ICU (Blake 10)

Proportion of Infants 22 to 29 Weeks Gestation Screened for Retinopathy of Prematurity (ROP)								
Fiscal Year/Quarter	2010 Q4	2011 Q1	2011 Q2	2011 Q3	2011 Q4	2012 Q1	2012 Q2	2012 Q3
Reporting Period	Jul - Sep 2010	Oct - Dec 2010	Jan - Mar 2011	Apr - Jun 2011	Jul - Sep 2011	Oct - Dec 2011	Jan - Mar 2012	Apr - Jun 2012
Neonatal ICU (Blake 10)	100.00%	100.00%	100.00%	100.00%	100.00%	100.00%	100.00%	100.00%
Vermont Oxford Network (VON) Benchmark*	93.80%	93.80%	93.80%	93.80%	93.80%	93.80%	93.80%	93.80%

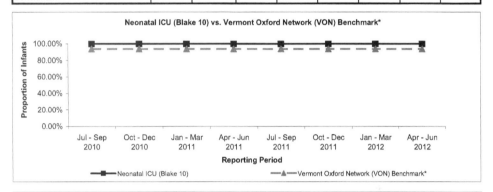

Proportion of Infants 22 to 29 Weeks Gestation with Retinopathy of Prematurity (Stages 1- 5)								
Fiscal Year/Quarter	2010 Q4	2011 Q1	2011 Q2	2011 Q3	2011 Q4	2012 Q1	2012 Q2	2012 Q3
Reporting Period	Jul - Sep 2010	Oct - Dec 2010	Jan - Mar 2011	Apr - Jun 2011	Jul - Sep 2011	Oct - Dec 2011	Jan - Mar 2012	Apr - Jun 2012
Neonatal ICU (Blake 10)	33.33%	0.00%	0.00%	11.11%	0.00%	8.33%	0.00%	22.22%
Vermont Oxford Network (VON) Benchmark*	43.20%	43.20%	43.20%	43.20%	43.20%	43.20%	43.20%	43.20%

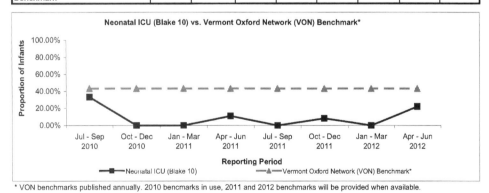

* VON benchmarks published annually. 2010 bencmarks in use, 2011 and 2012 benchmarks will be provided when available.

FIGURE C.1

MGHfC NICU and VON ROP rates for 2010 through Q2 2012.

Index

hospital-acquired pressure ulcers
(HAPUs), 27
Hotline, 51

I
image of nursing, 194
implementation models
evidence-based practice (EBP), 79–80
innovation, 114. *See also* innovation
individual development plans (IDPs), 149
infrastructure, 17–19
Institute for Patient Care (IPC), 19–20
centers within, 22–26
goal implementation, 21–22
outcomes of, 26–35
research, 127–128. *See also* research
innovation, 106–109
creation of innovative processes,
110–113
definition of, 106
development of products, 109–110
evaluation of, 114–123
Professional Practice Model (PPM),
162
unit evaluation design, 118–120
Innovation Unit Initiative (IU), 115–122
inquiry (culture of), 1–2
agendas for change, 2–5
care delivery integration, 5–7
learning environments, 7–11
Institute for Healthcare Improvement
(IHI), 97, 110–111, 112
Institute for Nursing Healthcare
Leadership (INHL), 2010, 175
Institute for Patient Care (IPC), 19–20,
22–26, 39
Center for Innovations in Care
Delivery, 25
goals of, 19, 21–22

Maxwell & Eleanor Blum Patient &
Family Learning Center, 24
Norman Knight Nursing Center for
Clinical & Professional Development,
22–24
outcomes of, 26–35
priorities of, 20
Yvonne L. Munn Center for Nursing
Research, 25–26, 40–41
Institute of Medicine (IOM), 17, 75
Value and Science-Driven Health
Care, 78
Institutional Review Board (IRB), 47, 199
membership in, 130–131
intensive care units (ICUs), 233
interdisciplinary relationships, 194
interdisciplinary teams, 241–245
international influence, Institute for
Patient Care (IPC), 33–34
International Nursing Review, 183, 186
Iowa Model of Evidence-Based Practice to
Promote Quality Care, 80
Ives Erickson, Jeanette, 40

J
Jones, Dorothy A., 8, 9
The Journal for Nurse Practitioners, 184
Journal for Nurses in Staff Development,
185
Journal of Advanced Nursing, 184
Journal of Clinical Nursing, 186
*Journal of Continuing Education in
Nursing*, 187
Journal of Gerontological Nursing, 184
*Journal of Hospice & Palliative Care
Nursing*, 186
Journal of Nursing Education, 184
journals, 156

2014
American Journal of Nursing
Book *of the* Year

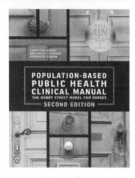

First Place

Community/Public Health

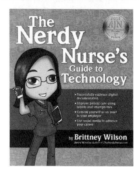

First Place

Information Technology/
Social Media

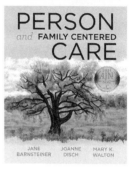

First Place

Nursing Management/
Leadership

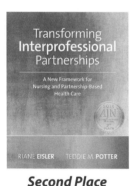

Second Place

Professional Development
and Issues

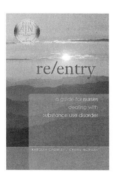

First Place
Two Categories

History and Public Policy
and
Professional Development
and Issues

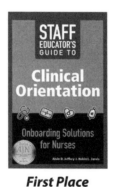

First Place

Nursing Education/
Continuing Education

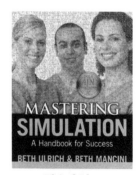

Third Place

Information Technology/
Social Media

Learn more at **www.nursingknowledge.org/sttibooks**.
Discounts are available for institutional purchases.
Call **888.NKI.4.YOU** for details.

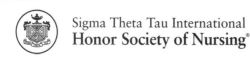

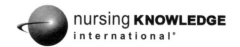

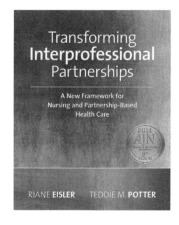
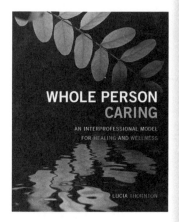
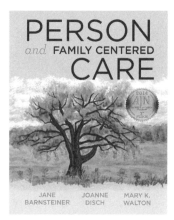
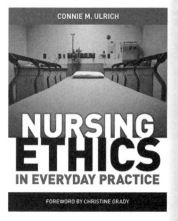
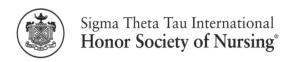
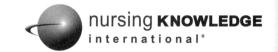

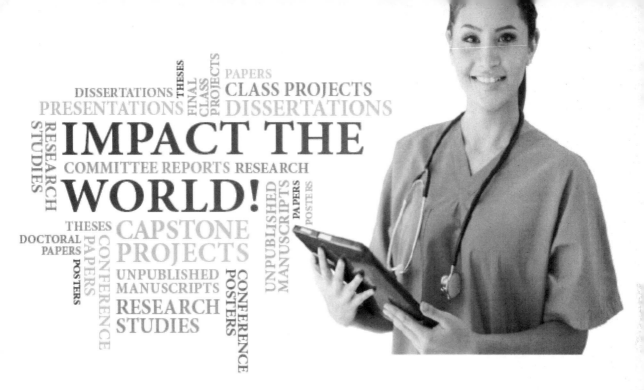

THREE Ways to Impact the World of Nursing With the Virginia Henderson Global Nursing e-Repository

1. Nurses and students may self-archive full-text items including research studies, reports, posters, unpublished manuscripts, and more. All items are peer-reviewed.

2. Schools of nursing may request a collection or collections to showcase students' work at the graduate and undergraduate levels.

3. National and international nursing organizations may request a collection to share their corporately authored documents such as best-practice guidelines, committee reports, and position papers.

For details about this free resource available to members and nonmembers of the Honor Society of Nursing, Sigma Theta Tau International, view the instructions and guidelines on the website and then contact Kimberly Thompson, MLS, repository manager, at repository@stti.org.

www.nursingrepository.org

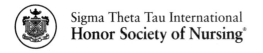

Sigma Theta Tau International
Honor Society of Nursing

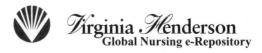

Virginia Henderson
Global Nursing e-Repository

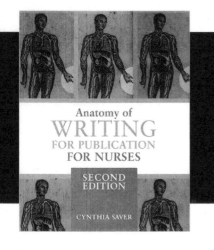
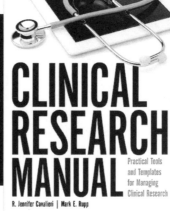
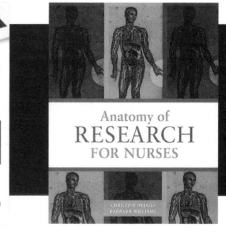

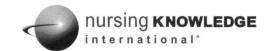